NHA Certified Phlebotomy Technician Practice Exam 160 Questions & Answers Explanation

I0465397

Disclaimer:

The information provided in this book, including but not limited to the questions, answers, explanations, and study material, is intended for educational purposes only. While every effort has been made to ensure its accuracy and completeness, the publisher and authors make no warranties or representations, express or implied, regarding the content's reliability, suitability, or applicability for any particular purpose.

The content provided in this book is not intended to replace professional advice or guidance, and readers are encouraged to consult with qualified professionals or relevant authorities regarding certification-related matters.

The publisher and authors shall not be held liable for any damages, losses, or liabilities arising from the use of this publication, including but not limited to direct, indirect, incidental, punitive, or consequential damages.

Contents

Book Introduction

Preparing for the NHA Certified Phlebotomy Technician (CPT) exam can be challenging, especially with the wide range of skills and knowledge areas covered. This practice exam book offers 160 meticulously crafted questions that cover each critical domain of the CPT exam, including anatomy and physiology, specimen collection, safety and compliance, patient interaction, and handling and processing samples. Each question is accompanied by a detailed answer explanation, ensuring that you not only know the correct answer but understand the reasoning behind it.

The book is designed for both new phlebotomy candidates and seasoned healthcare professionals seeking to brush up on their knowledge. By studying these questions, candidates can gain confidence, reinforce their understanding of key topics, and improve their test-taking strategies.

Exam Coverage:

- **Patient Preparation and Safety**: Proper patient identification, consent, and safety protocols

- **Blood Collection Procedures**: Venipuncture, capillary puncture, and special collection procedures

- **Specimen Handling and Processing**: Sample storage, labeling, and transportation protocols

- **Infection Control**: Techniques for maintaining a sterile environment and preventing contamination

- **Anatomy and Physiology**: Focus on circulatory system knowledge relevant to phlebotomy

CERTIFIED PHLEBOTOMY TECHNICIAN [CPT] EXAM 160 QUESTIONS

Anatomy and Physiology

1. A medical assistant is preparing to perform venipuncture on a patient. After assessing the patient's veins, the assistant notices that the basilic and cephalic veins are both visible but may not offer the best access due to their location and proximity to arteries and nerves. Given this assessment, which vein would be the most appropriate to use for venipuncture, considering

the balance of safety, accessibility, and comfort for the patient?

A) Basilic vein

B) Median cubital vein

C) Cephalic vein

D) Femoral vein

2. Erythrocytes play a crucial role in maintaining the body's physiological functions. Comprising approximately 40-45% of blood volume, these specialized cells perform a function vital to cellular metabolism and overall homeostasis. Hemoglobin, the oxygen-carrying protein within erythrocytes, enables the transport of gases essential for life. Considering their structural adaptations and functional importance, what is the primary function of erythrocytes in the human circulatory system?

A) To defend the body against pathogens by engulfing and destroying foreign invaders

B) To transport nutrients such as glucose and amino acids to the body's tissues

C) To transport oxygen from the lungs to tissues and carry carbon dioxide back to the lungs

D) To initiate the clotting process by releasing clotting factors at the site of injury

3. The regulation of blood pH is a complex process involving multiple organ systems. Which of the following systems is primarily responsible for the long-term regulation of blood pH by adjusting hydrogen ion concentration and bicarbonate reabsorption?

A) **Respiratory system**, by modulating carbon dioxide exhalation and influencing the carbonic acid-bicarbonate buffer system

B) **Urinary system**, through renal mechanisms that control the excretion of hydrogen ions (H+) and the reabsorption of bicarbonate (HCO3-)

C) **Endocrine system**, by releasing hormones that control blood pH and electrolyte balance

D) **Cardiovascular system**, through the regulation of blood flow and the transport of acids and bases to the kidneys and lungs for processing

4. A patient presents with symptoms of heart failure, including fatigue, shortness of breath, and fluid retention. Upon further examination and imaging, it is noted that the heart's ability to contract is diminished. Understanding that the heart is composed of multiple layers, which layer of the heart is primarily responsible for generating the force necessary for its pumping action, and how does damage to this layer contribute to the patient's symptoms?

A) Endocardium
B) Myocardium
C) Epicardium
D) Pericardium

5. The circulatory system includes various blood vessels that transport blood between the heart and the lungs to maintain oxygen and carbon dioxide balance. After oxygen is absorbed in the lungs, it must be delivered back to the heart for systemic distribution. Which of the following

blood vessels is responsible for carrying *oxygenated blood* from the lungs to the heart?

A) Pulmonary artery

B) Aorta

C) Pulmonary vein

D) Superior vena cava

6. Gas exchange within the respiratory system is a finely regulated process that occurs at the microscopic level. Which of the following structures is the primary site of gas exchange, characterized by its thin epithelial walls, extensive capillary network, and large surface area designed to facilitate the diffusion of oxygen and carbon dioxide?

A) **Trachea**, which functions primarily as the main airway for air conduction to the lungs

B) **Bronchi**, responsible for conducting air deeper into the lungs and distributing it to the lobes

C) **Alveoli**, specialized for efficient gas exchange due to their thin walls and proximity to pulmonary capillaries

D) **Bronchioles**, smaller airways responsible for controlling airflow resistance and the distribution of air to terminal structures

7. The initiation of the clotting process is a complex physiological response involving the interaction of cellular components and biochemical factors. Which of the following blood cell types are primarily responsible for initiating the coagulation cascade by adhering to damaged blood vessels and releasing chemicals that activate clotting factors?

A) **Erythrocytes**, which carry oxygen and assist in the transport of clotting factors to the site of injury

B) **Leukocytes**, which initiate the clotting process through the release of inflammatory cytokines during injury

C) **Platelets**, which adhere to the site of vascular injury, release thromboxane, and promote fibrin formation

D) **Plasma cells**, which synthesize and release

antibodies involved in the inflammatory phase of hemostasis

8. The cerebral cortex, specifically the motor cortex located in the frontal lobe, is primarily responsible for controlling voluntary muscle movements, while the spinal cord is mainly responsible for reflex actions.

A. True

B. False

9. The component of blood primarily responsible for the body's immune response is _____, which functions by identifying and attacking foreign invaders. This component is crucial for protecting the body against infections.

A) Red blood cells (RBCs)

B) Platelets

C) Plasma

D) White blood cells (WBCs)

10. The process of hemostasis involves vascular spasm, platelet plug formation, and coagulation, but does not include clot retraction or fibrinolysis.

A) True

B) False

11. The blood type that is known as the universal donor, because it can be safely transfused to individuals of any blood type without causing an immune reaction, is _____.

A) Type A

B) Type B

C) Type AB

D) Type O

12. A patient presents with swelling in the legs and ankles, and upon further investigation, the physician suspects a malfunction in the lymphatic system. Considering the interconnectedness of the lymphatic and circulatory systems, which of the following functions of the lymphatic system is most crucial in preventing this type of fluid accumulation, and how does the dysfunction of this system contribute to the patient's symptoms?

A) Transporting oxygen and nutrients to tissues
B) Regulating blood glucose and nutrient absorption
C) Returning excess interstitial fluid to the bloodstream
D) Producing immune cells to fight infection

13. Platelets, also known as thrombocytes, are small, disc-shaped components of blood. These cells play an essential role in the body's response to injury, particularly in maintaining hemostasis and wound repair. When an injury occurs, platelets are activated and contribute to preventing excessive blood loss. Considering this,

what is the main function of platelets in the blood?

A) To transport oxygen from the lungs to tissues

B) To produce antibodies and defend the body against pathogens

C) To initiate blood clot formation to prevent excessive bleeding

D) To remove waste products from the tissues to the kidneys for filtration

14. The liver plays a crucial role in maintaining homeostasis by filtering and detoxifying the blood. Which of the following accurately describes the liver's role in detoxification, including the processes involved in metabolizing toxins and drugs?

A) **Kidneys**, which filter the blood through glomerular filtration and remove waste products primarily in the form of urine

B) **Liver**, which detoxifies the blood via enzymatic pathways such as cytochrome P450, converting lipophilic toxins into hydrophilic compounds for excretion

C) **Spleen**, which is involved in immune surveillance and the filtration of damaged red blood cells from circulation

D) **Pancreas**, which assists in blood detoxification by regulating blood sugar levels and producing digestive enzymes

15. Hemoglobin is a crucial protein found in red blood cells (erythrocytes) that enables these cells to carry out their primary function in the circulatory system. Given its specific molecular structure and interaction with gases, what is the main role of hemoglobin in red blood cells?

A) To transport nutrients like glucose and fatty acids to tissues

B) To transport oxygen from the lungs to tissues and carbon dioxide from tissues to the lungs

C) To initiate the process of blood clotting at the site of injury

D) To regulate the body's pH by neutralizing acids in the bloodstream

16. A patient presents with malnutrition and weight loss despite a regular diet. Upon examination, the physician suspects a dysfunction in the digestive system. Considering the various components of the digestive system, which specific part is primarily responsible for the absorption of nutrients, and how might impairment in this part contribute to the patient's symptoms of malnutrition and weight loss?

A) Stomach
B) Small intestine
C) Large intestine
D) Esophagus

17. Which of the following hormones regulates blood glucose levels by promoting the uptake of glucose into cells?

A) Glucagon
B) Insulin
C) Adrenaline
D) Cortisol

18. The structure in the heart responsible for initiating the heartbeat by generating electrical impulses that regulate the heart's rhythm is the _____.

A) Atrioventricular (AV) node

B) Bundle of His

C) Sinoatrial (SA) node

D) Purkinje fibers

19. The primary function of the large intestine is to absorb nutrients from digested food and to produce digestive enzymes.

A) True
B) False

20. Which structure in the brain is responsible for regulating vital functions such as heart rate, blood pressure, and respiration?

A) Cerebellum

B) Medulla oblongata

C) Hypothalamus

D) Thalamus

Medical Terminology in Phlebotomy

21. The process of blood clotting, which is essential for preventing excessive blood loss after an injury, is known as _____.

A) Hemolysis

B) Hemostasis

C) Coagulation

D) Erythropoiesis

22. A patient presents with recurrent infections and a complete blood count (CBC) reveals a significantly low white blood cell count. In the context of the immune response, which term describes this decrease in white blood cells, and what are the potential clinical implications of this condition for the patient's health and infection risk?

A) Leukocytosis

B) Leukopenia

C) Thrombocytopenia

D) Anemia

23. The term "hematocrit" is often used in clinical settings as an important measure in assessing a patient's blood. It provides valuable information about the proportion of different components in the blood and can indicate various medical conditions. What does the term "hematocrit" refer to?

A) The percentage of white blood cells in the blood

B) The percentage of red blood cells in the blood

C) The concentration of hemoglobin in the blood

D) The ratio of plasma to total blood volume

24. Medical terminology often uses specific suffixes and prefixes to describe different conditions related to the body's anatomy and physiology. The term that indicates inflammation of a vein is used to describe conditions that affect venous structures, leading to symptoms like pain, swelling, and redness. Which of the following medical terms refers to the inflammation of a vein?

A) Phlebitis

B) Thrombosis

C) Vasculitis

D) Arteritis

Aseptic Techniques

25. During a routine venipuncture, it is critical to minimize the risk of infection at the site of needle

insertion. Which antiseptic is considered the standard for this procedure, and what are the key properties that make it suitable for skin disinfection prior to venipuncture?

A) Hydrogen peroxide

B) Iodine-based solution

C) 70% Isopropyl alcohol

D) Chlorhexidine gluconate

26. Why is it important to allow the antiseptic to dry completely before performing venipuncture?

A) It ensures maximum effectiveness in killing microorganisms

B) It prevents contamination of the needle

C) It reduces the risk of patient discomfort

D) It avoids the mixing of antiseptic with the blood sample

27. Venipuncture is a common medical procedure used to draw blood or administer intravenous therapy. Before performing venipuncture,

healthcare professionals typically apply antiseptics to the puncture site. What is the primary purpose of using antiseptics during venipuncture?

A) To reduce pain and discomfort during the procedure

B) To prevent blood from clotting at the puncture site

C) To destroy or inhibit microorganisms and prevent infection

D) To improve blood flow to the area for easier access to the vein

28. In the context of phlebotomy, maintaining aseptic technique is critical to preventing infections and ensuring patient safety. Which of the following actions is considered a breach of aseptic technique, and what is the underlying rationale for this standard?

A) **Wearing sterile gloves** throughout the procedure to minimize contamination from the healthcare worker's hands

B) **Cleansing the puncture site with an alcohol swab** to reduce microbial load and prevent infection at the site of entry

C) **Palpating the puncture site with bare hands after cleansing,** which could introduce contaminants and negate the antiseptic effect

D) **Immediately disposing of the used needle in a designated sharps container** to prevent needlestick injuries and further contamination

29. During a blood culture collection, what additional step should be taken to ensure aseptic technique compared to routine venipuncture?

A) Use a sterile gauze to wipe the puncture site

B) Use both alcohol and povidone-iodine to cleanse the site

C) Re-clean the site immediately after needle insertion

D) Use 70% isopropyl alcohol only

30. In preparing for a venipuncture procedure, maintaining aseptic conditions is crucial to

prevent infection. What is the minimum recommended duration for handwashing, and what key factors contribute to the effectiveness of this practice in a clinical setting?

A) 10 seconds

B) 20 seconds

C) 30 seconds

D) 1 minute

31. In phlebotomy, the choice between sterile and non-sterile gloves is influenced by specific patient conditions and the potential risks involved. Considering the implications for patient safety and infection control, which of the following scenarios necessitates the use of sterile gloves, and what are the potential consequences of not adhering to this practice?

A) Performing venipuncture on a healthy adult— Assess the risks of using non-sterile gloves in this context and the importance of maintaining standard precautions.

B) Collecting blood from a patient with an active

infection Evaluate why sterile gloves are critical in this scenario and the potential for pathogen transmission if non-sterile gloves are used.

C) **Drawing blood for routine laboratory tests**— Discuss the rationale for using non-sterile gloves and how this aligns with typical infection control measures.

D) **Conducting a fingerstick blood test on a pediatric patient**—Analyze the appropriateness of non-sterile gloves in this situation and any considerations that may warrant the use of sterile gloves.

32. Aseptic techniques are critical in phlebotomy to prevent infection and ensure patient safety. One key practice involves the use of gloves throughout the procedure. What is the primary reason for wearing gloves during the entire phlebotomy procedure?

A) To improve grip on the needle and other equipment

B) To protect the healthcare worker from exposure

to bloodborne pathogens

C) To keep the puncture site warm during the procedure

D) To ensure that the blood sample is not contaminated by skin flora

33. A phlebotomist is preparing to perform a venipuncture on a patient. To ensure the procedure is conducted under optimal aseptic conditions and to minimize the risk of infection, which practice should the phlebotomist follow regarding skin preparation, and why is this practice essential for patient safety?

A) By using a tourniquet only to visualize the vein

B) By applying an antiseptic solution and allowing it to dry completely

C) By wiping the area with a dry gauze to remove any visible dirt

D) By asking the patient to wash the site with soap and water before the procedure

34. In venipuncture procedures, the choice of vein is crucial for successful blood collection. Which of the following veins, located in the antecubital fossa, is most commonly selected for venipuncture due to its anatomical features and accessibility?

A) **Cephalic vein**, which runs along the lateral aspect of the forearm and is more variable in size, often leading to difficulty in access

B) **Basilic vein**, positioned on the medial side of the arm, which can be challenging to access due to its proximity to nerves and deeper location

C) **Median cubital vein**, the preferred site for venipuncture because of its central location, size, and minimal risk of complications with surrounding structures

D) **Radial vein**, typically found in the wrist area, which is not commonly used for venipuncture due to its smaller diameter and depth

35. When selecting a vein for venipuncture, the phlebotomist encounters a patient with a higher body mass index (BMI). Which of the following factors makes the cephalic vein a favorable choice in this situation, and what considerations should the phlebotomist keep in mind regarding this vein's anatomical location and accessibility?

A) It is the largest vein in the body, allowing for higher blood flow.

B) It is often more visible and easier to palpate in obese patients, facilitating access.

C) It is located closer to the heart, ensuring better sample quality.

D) It has a direct connection to the jugular vein, reducing complications during collection.

36. Understanding the anatomy of the veins in the antecubital fossa is essential for healthcare professionals performing venipuncture. Among the veins in this area, the basilic vein and the median cubital vein have specific locations relative to one another. Which of the following

statements accurately describes the location of the basilic vein in relation to the median cubital vein?

A) The basilic vein is located medial to the median cubital vein.

B) The basilic vein is located lateral to the median cubital vein.

C) The basilic vein is located posterior to the median cubital vein.

D) The basilic vein and median cubital vein are located in the same anatomical plane.

37. When performing venipuncture, healthcare professionals must be aware of the anatomical considerations and potential risks associated with accessing specific veins. The basilic vein, while often used, poses certain risks compared to other veins. What is the primary risk associated with puncturing the basilic vein during venipuncture?

A) Increased risk of puncturing an artery

B) Higher likelihood of nerve damage

C) Greater chance of hematoma formation

D) Difficulty in locating the vein

38. When considering venipuncture on the foot, several factors influence the choice of vein to minimize complications and ensure successful blood collection. Which vein is most commonly selected for this purpose, and what considerations should be taken into account regarding anatomical location and potential risks?

A) **Dorsalis pedis vein**—Assess the advantages and disadvantages of using this vein, including its accessibility and the risks associated with accessing deeper structures.

B) **Great saphenous vein**—Evaluate why this vein is preferred for venipuncture in the foot, considering its size, location, and the lower risk of complications compared to other veins.

C) **Lateral plantar vein**—Discuss the characteristics of this vein and the potential complications that may arise when attempting venipuncture.

D) **Medial plantar vein**—Analyze the appropriateness of using this vein for blood collection and the anatomical considerations that may impact the procedure.

39. The median cubital vein is often the preferred site for venipuncture in clinical practice. Understanding the anatomical features of this vein can clarify why it is commonly selected. What is the primary anatomical reason that makes the median cubital vein the most commonly chosen site for venipuncture?

A) It is the largest vein in the antecubital fossa.

B) It is located centrally and is typically more superficial than other veins.

C) It has a larger lumen than the basilic vein.

D) It is directly connected to the brachial artery.

40. In the practice of phlebotomy, selecting the appropriate vein for venipuncture is crucial for both the success of the procedure and the comfort of the patient. Under which circumstances might a phlebotomist prefer to use the cephalic vein instead of the median cubital vein, and what

factors should be considered in this decision-making process?

A) **Patient anatomy**—Evaluate how variations in a patient's anatomy, such as obesity or previous venipuncture scars, might impact the visibility and accessibility of the median cubital vein compared to the cephalic vein.

B) **Patient history**—Discuss the implications of a patient's medical history, including clotting disorders or vascular diseases, and how these factors might influence the choice of vein for venipuncture.

C) **Volume and type of blood draw**—Analyze the significance of the volume of blood required for testing and whether this influences the decision to choose the cephalic vein over the median cubital vein.

D) **Patient comfort and anxiety**—Consider how a patient's level of anxiety or discomfort with needles may affect the choice of vein, including the potential impact of using the cephalic vein in certain populations.

41. The median antebrachial vein is an important structure in the forearm, particularly in the context of venipuncture. Understanding its anatomical significance can help healthcare professionals make informed decisions during blood draws. What is the anatomical significance of the median antebrachial vein during venipuncture?

A) It serves as a primary route for blood return to the heart.

B) It is a common site for venipuncture due to its large size.

C) It may serve as a connection between the basilic and cephalic veins, providing alternative access points.

D) It is located deep within the forearm, reducing the risk of complications.

42. In the practice of phlebotomy, careful selection of the venipuncture site is essential to minimize the risk of complications such as nerve damage or arterial puncture. Which of the

following anatomical considerations is most critical in ensuring patient safety during the procedure?

A) **The depth of the vein in relation to the skin surface**—Analyze how the depth can affect needle insertion and the potential for complications if a deeper vein is accessed incorrectly.

B) **The size and visibility of the vein**—Evaluate the importance of vein size and visibility in successful blood collection and the implications of choosing smaller veins.

C) **The proximity of major nerves and arteries to the chosen vein**—Discuss why understanding the anatomy of the area, particularly the location of major nerves and arteries, is vital for preventing complications.

D) **The patient's age and overall health status**—Consider how these factors can influence the selection of the venipuncture site and the potential risks involved in the procedure.

Blood Components

43. A laboratory technician is processing a blood sample for testing. When deciding whether to use plasma or serum for different diagnostic purposes, what is the primary biochemical distinction between the two, and how does this difference impact the type of tests that can be performed on each?

A) Plasma contains clotting factors, while serum does not, making plasma suitable for coagulation studies.

B) Serum contains white blood cells, while plasma does not, making serum ideal for cellular studies.

C) Plasma contains more nutrients than serum, making it preferable for metabolic analysis.

D) Serum is the liquid portion of blood, while plasma is the cellular portion, which determines its use in cellular diagnostics.

44. Platelets, also known as thrombocytes, are one of the key components of blood, alongside red blood cells and white blood cells. Understanding

their function is essential in comprehending the body's response to injury and blood loss. What role do platelets play in the blood?

A) They transport oxygen to tissues.
B) They help in the formation of blood clots to stop bleeding.
C) They fight infections by attacking bacteria and viruses.
D) They regulate the body's immune response.

45. The blood consists of various components, each playing a unique role in maintaining the body's health and functions. Among these components, one is primarily responsible for the body's immune response and fighting infections. Which component of blood is mainly involved in immune response and fighting infections?

A) Red blood cells
B) Platelets
C) Plasma
D) White blood cells

lymphocytes, monocytes, eosinophils, and basophils, each specializing in different aspects of the immune defense.

46. Centrifugation is a common laboratory technique used to separate blood components for analysis. When a blood sample is centrifuged, it divides into distinct layers based on the density of its components. In what order do these layers typically appear from top to bottom, and what clinical significance does each layer hold in terms of diagnosis and treatment?

A) **Plasma, buffy coat, red blood cells**—Discuss the composition of each layer, including the importance of plasma for testing electrolytes, proteins, and hormones, the role of the buffy coat in evaluating immune function, and how red blood cells reflect oxygen-carrying capacity and anemia.

B) **Buffy coat, plasma, red blood cells**—Evaluate why this order is not typically observed in a centrifuged sample and how misinterpretation of the layers could lead to diagnostic errors.

C) **Red blood cells, buffy coat, plasma**—Analyze the density gradient and explain why this order of separation occurs, focusing on the physical properties of blood components.

D) **Plasma, red blood cells, buffy coat**—Consider whether this configuration could indicate a pathological condition or an error in the centrifugation process.

47. In a normal adult, red blood cells (RBCs) are produced in the _____, where they develop and mature before being released into the bloodstream to transport oxygen.

A) Liver

B) Lymph nodes

C) Bone marrow

D) Spleen

48. The bicarbonate buffering system is the primary mechanism for maintaining blood pH

balance, and it functions without interaction from other physiological systems.

A) True

B) False

49. What does the term "plasma" refer to in a blood sample that has been treated with an anticoagulant?

A. The liquid portion of the blood that contains clotting factors

B. The liquid portion of the blood that is free of all proteins

C. The cellular components separated after centrifugation

D. The fluid part of the blood after it has clotted

50. A clinician is preparing a blood sample for testing and must decide between using plasma or serum. Given the biochemical composition of these components, which of the following is not

found in serum, and why is its absence important for specific types of diagnostic tests?

A) Electrolytes, which are crucial for balancing body fluids

B) Antibodies, which help in immune response diagnostics

C) Clotting factors, which are required for coagulation tests

D) Hormones, which are vital for assessing endocrine function

51. Certain medical conditions are associated with abnormal levels of red blood cells. One of these conditions involves an elevated number of red blood cells in the bloodstream, leading to increased blood viscosity. Which of the following conditions is characterized by an elevated number of red blood cells?

A) Anemia

B) Leukocytosis

C) Polycythemia

D) Thrombocytopenia

52. Neutrophils are one of the most abundant types of white blood cells and play a critical role in the body's defense mechanism. Understanding their specific function is key to grasping how the immune system responds to infections. What is the primary function of neutrophils in the blood?

A) To produce antibodies to fight infections

B) To initiate the clotting process in response to injury

C) To engulf and destroy bacteria and other pathogens

D) To transport oxygen to tissues

53. In the complex process of hemostasis, fibrin plays a crucial role in the stabilization of blood clots. How does fibrin contribute to the final stages of clot formation, and what clinical significance does this function have in preventing excessive blood loss?

A) To initiate the formation of platelets—Evaluate why the process of platelet formation is not associated with fibrin's role and how platelet aggregation occurs before fibrin involvement.

B) To dissolve blood clots once healing is complete—Analyze how fibrin's function differs from that of fibrinolysis, the process responsible for clot breakdown.

C) To form a mesh that stabilizes the platelet plug—Discuss the transformation of fibrinogen into fibrin, how it creates a mesh-like network, and its importance in reinforcing the platelet plug to prevent blood loss.

D) To activate clotting factors in the blood—Examine how clotting factors are activated prior to fibrin's involvement and how fibrin's role is downstream in the clotting cascade.

54. The prothrombin time (PT) test is used to evaluate the intrinsic and common coagulation pathways, and an elevated PT can indicate issues such as liver disease, vitamin K deficiency, or the effects of anticoagulant therapy.

A) True

B) False

55. In clinical settings, understanding the spleen's function is essential, especially when assessing patients with hemolytic disorders or conditions that affect red blood cell turnover. What specific role does the spleen play in the lifecycle of red blood cells, and why is this function critical to overall hematological health?

A) It produces red blood cells in adults, ensuring adequate oxygen transport during stress.

B) It stores excess red blood cells, releasing them during hemorrhagic emergencies to maintain blood volume.

C) It filters and removes old or damaged red blood cells, recycling iron and preventing accumulation of dysfunctional cells.

D) It converts red blood cells into white blood cells, contributing to immune response regulation.

56. Platelets, or thrombocytes, play a critical role in blood clotting. However, abnormal increases in platelet counts, known as thrombocytosis, can impact the body in various ways. How does a high platelet count (thrombocytosis) affect the body?

A) It leads to excessive bleeding and bruising.

B) It increases the risk of abnormal blood clot formation.

C) It causes a reduction in white blood cell production.

D) It decreases oxygen transport to tissues.

57. White blood cells are crucial components of the immune system, with different types playing distinct roles. In the case of allergic reactions and asthma, a particular type of white blood cell is predominantly involved in the inflammatory response. Which type of white blood cell is most commonly associated with allergic reactions and asthma?

A) Neutrophils

B) Eosinophils

C) Lymphocytes

D) Monocytes

Blood Group Systems

58. Blood group systems are classified based on the presence or absence of specific antigens on the surface of red blood cells. These antigens play a critical role in determining compatibility for blood transfusions and organ transplants. Which of the following blood group systems is determined by the presence or absence of antigens on the surface of red blood cells?

A) ABO system

B) Rh system

C) HLA system

D) MHC system

59. In addition to the ABO blood group system, the Rh factor plays a crucial role in determining blood transfusion compatibility. Understanding the significance of the Rh factor is vital for safe transfusion practices. What is the primary purpose of the Rh factor in blood transfusion compatibility?

A) It determines the ability of blood to clot.

B) It affects whether a blood transfusion will result in an immune reaction.

C) It regulates the oxygen-carrying capacity of red blood cells.

D) It helps identify whether the blood type is A, B, AB, or O.

60. In clinical practice, understanding blood compatibility is crucial for safe transfusion procedures. A patient with AB positive blood type is considered the universal recipient. Which of the following blood types can they safely receive, and what immunological mechanisms make this possible?

A) **O positive and O negative only**—Discuss the significance of type O blood in transfusion practices and why these blood types are compatible with most patients.

B) **A positive and B positive only**—Evaluate the rationale behind limiting transfusions to these specific blood types and the role of Rh factor in this scenario.

C) **AB positive only**—Analyze why restricting transfusions to only AB positive donors would be unnecessarily limiting and how this could affect patient outcomes.

D) **All blood types**—Explain why AB positive patients are considered universal recipients, focusing on the absence of anti-A, anti-B, and anti-Rh antibodies, and the immunological compatibility with all blood types.

61. A patient with type O negative blood can only receive blood from donors with _____, because their blood lacks A, B, and Rh antigens, making them susceptible to immune reactions if given other blood types.

A) Type A positive blood

B) Type O negative blood

C) Type O positive blood

D) Any blood type

62. The Rh system, which involves the Rh factor (also known as Rhesus factor), is critical in blood typing and is used to determine whether a person's blood type is Rh-positive or Rh-negative. Rh-positive individuals have the Rh antigen on their red blood cells, while Rh-negative individuals do not have this antigen.

A) True
B) False

63. Blood group systems are essential for determining compatibility in blood transfusions. While several systems are widely used, not all blood group systems are commonly applied in transfusion medicine. Which of the following is

NOT a common blood group system used in blood transfusions?

A) ABO

B) Rh

C) HLA

D) Kell

64. Crossmatching is a crucial step in ensuring the safety of blood transfusions. When conducting a crossmatch test, which of the following is the most critical consideration to prevent hemolytic reactions, and why?

A) **Ensuring the donor blood is free from infections**—Consider why screening for infectious diseases, while essential, is not the primary concern in crossmatching specifically.

B) **Ensuring the patient and donor blood types are compatible**—Analyze how the compatibility of ABO and Rh antigens plays a pivotal role in avoiding dangerous transfusion reactions, and discuss the implications of undetected incompatibilities.

C) **Confirming the patient's medical history and previous transfusions**—Evaluate how a patient's transfusion history, while important, is supplementary to the immediate compatibility of the current donor and recipient blood.

D) **Matching the Rh factor of the donor and recipient**—Discuss the role of the Rh factor and why it is a significant but not exclusive consideration in the broader context of the crossmatch process.

65. Blood transfusions must be carefully matched to prevent dangerous immune responses. If a patient with type B positive blood receives type A positive blood, what type of reaction is most likely to occur?

A) No reaction, as both are Rh-positive

B) Hemolytic transfusion reaction

C) Delayed allergic reaction

D) Immune tolerance due to shared antigens

66. The Kell blood group system is one of several blood group systems important in transfusion

modioino. Underotanding its role is critical for ensuring safe blood transfusions. Which statement best describes the role of the Kell blood group system in transfusion medicine?

A) It is the primary system used for determining blood type compatibility.

B) It can lead to hemolytic transfusion reactions if incompatible blood is transfused.

C) It has no impact on pregnancy and fetal health.

D) It is only relevant for organ transplantation, not blood transfusions.

67. A mother with type A negative blood has a newborn with type A positive blood. This scenario raises specific concerns regarding the newborn's health. What is the most likely risk, and what interventions are commonly used to prevent this condition?

A) **ABO incompatibility**—Consider the likelihood of ABO incompatibility and its typical effects in this mother-baby pairing, and why this would be less of a concern compared to Rh issues.

B) **Rh incompatibility**—Discuss the mechanism of Rh incompatibility, focusing on how the Rh-negative mother's immune system may produce antibodies against the Rh-positive baby's red blood cells, leading to hemolytic disease of the newborn (HDN), and the role of RhoGAM in preventing this condition.

C) **Hemophilia**—Evaluate why hemophilia, a genetic bleeding disorder, is unrelated to the blood types and Rh status of the mother and baby.

D) **Iron deficiency anemia**—Analyze how iron deficiency anemia could occur in newborns but is not specifically linked to maternal-fetal blood type differences.

68. If a patient with type B negative blood receives a transfusion of type B positive blood, their immune system is likely to produce antibodies against the _____, potentially leading to an immune reaction.

A) A antigen

B) B antigen

C) Rh factor

D) Plasma proteins

69. A pregnant patient undergoes routine blood screening, and it is discovered that she has developed anti-K antibodies. Given the role of Kell antigens in the blood group system, what potential risks could this pose to her pregnancy, and how might this influence the management of her prenatal care and transfusion decisions?

A) The patient is at risk of developing hemolytic disease of the fetus and newborn (HDFN) if the fetus expresses the K antigen, requiring close monitoring.

B) The patient may experience a severe allergic reaction to transfusions with Rh-positive blood, necessitating the use of Rh-negative donors.

C) The presence of anti-K antibodies will only affect the ABO blood group compatibility in transfusions and has no impact on the pregnancy.

D) The fetus is at risk of developing severe anemia if maternal anti-K antibodies are not treated, requiring fetal blood transfusions early in the pregnancy.

70. The ABO blood group system is unique not only in its classification of blood types but also in the presence of naturally occurring antibodies. Which of the following statements is true regarding the ABO blood group system in relation to naturally occurring antibodies?

A) Individuals with type O blood have no naturally occurring antibodies.

B) Type A individuals have anti-B antibodies present in their plasma.

C) Type AB individuals have both anti-A and anti-B antibodies.

D) Type B individuals do not have any antibodies against A antigens.

71. In blood typing tests, specific reagents are used to identify the presence of antigens on red blood cells. Which reagent is utilized to detect A antigens, and what is the underlying mechanism of this test?

A) **Anti-B serum**—Evaluate why this reagent is inappropriate for detecting A antigens and discuss its role in identifying B antigens.

B) **Anti-A serum**—Discuss how this reagent interacts with A antigens on the red blood cell surface and the significance of agglutination in confirming blood type.

C) **Rho(D) immune globulin**—Analyze the purpose of this reagent in the context of Rh factor management rather than ABO typing.

D) **Antibody control serum**—Consider the role of control sera in blood typing and why they are not specific to any antigen detection.

72. A crossmatch test is an important procedure performed before blood transfusions to ensure compatibility between the donor's and recipient's blood. What is the primary goal of a crossmatch test?

A) To determine the donor's blood type only.

B) To check for the presence of infectious diseases in the donor blood.

C) To assess the compatibility between the donor's red blood cells and the recipient's plasma.

D) To evaluate the volume of blood needed for the transfusion.

73. In cases where an Rh-negative mother is pregnant with an Rh-positive baby, there is a risk of Rh incompatibility, which can lead to serious complications. What treatment may be given to the mother to prevent these complications?

A) Blood transfusion

B) Rho(D) immune globulin (RhIg)

C) Antibiotics

D) Anticoagulants

Capillary Puncture

74. When performing a capillary puncture, several factors can influence the accuracy of test

results. Which of the following is the most important factor to ensure accurate test results?

A) The choice of puncture site

B) The depth of the puncture

C) Proper warming of the site prior to puncture

D) The angle of the puncture

75. Capillary puncture is commonly performed on infants for blood sampling, and the appropriate depth is crucial to avoid complications. Which of the following best describes the appropriate depth for a capillary puncture on an infant?

A) 1-2 mm

B) 2-3 mm

C) 3-4 mm

D) 4-5 mm

76. A pediatric nurse is preparing to collect a blood sample from an infant and must choose between a heelstick and a fingerstick.

Considering the anatomical and developmental differences in infants compared to adults, which of the following is the most important reason for selecting a heelstick over a fingerstick for this age group, and how does this decision impact the infant's safety?

A) The heel contains more capillary-rich areas, making it the preferred site for collecting an adequate blood sample quickly and efficiently.

B) The skin on an infant's finger is more sensitive and prone to irritation, which could lead to excessive pain and discomfort during blood collection.

C) The risk of damaging the nerves in the finger is higher in infants, making the heelstick a safer option that reduces the risk of long-term nerve injury.

D) The pain receptors in the heel are less developed than in the fingers, which ensures the infant feels minimal pain during the procedure.

77. Capillary punctures, while generally safe and useful for obtaining blood samples, can sometimes lead to complications. Which of the

following is a common complication associated with capillary punctures?

A) Hematoma formation
B) Anaphylactic reaction
C) Systemic infection
D) Severe allergic reaction

78. When performing a capillary puncture on older children and adults, selecting the appropriate finger is crucial for obtaining a good blood sample while minimizing discomfort. Which finger is most commonly used for this procedure, and what factors influence this choice?

A) **Index finger**—Discuss the benefits and potential drawbacks of using the index finger compared to other fingers, particularly in terms of blood flow and sensitivity.

B) **Middle finger**—Analyze why the middle finger is typically preferred for capillary puncture, considering anatomical factors such as blood flow, size, and patient comfort.

C) **Ring finger**—Evaluate the considerations regarding using the ring finger, including potential complications and patient preferences, especially in individuals with frequent use of their hands.

D) **Thumb**—Examine why the thumb is generally avoided for capillary punctures, focusing on anatomical and functional reasons that could affect the quality of the sample and patient comfort.

79. During a capillary puncture procedure, it is acceptable to puncture the same site multiple times if the initial puncture does not yield an adequate sample or if there are complications.

A) True

B) False

80. Capillary puncture is the preferred method for obtaining blood samples when the patient has _____, making venipuncture challenging or unnecessary.

A) Normal hydration levels

B) Fragile veins or is a young child

C) The need for large volumes of blood

D) A requirement for blood culture testing

81. Certain conditions can render a capillary puncture site unsuitable for blood collection. Which of the following conditions would make a capillary puncture site unsuitable?

A) Presence of a rash or skin infection
B) Recent immunizations on the same arm
C) The patient's age
D) Presence of hair on the skin

82. When performing a capillary puncture, healthcare providers often choose this method for various types of blood tests. What type of blood is primarily obtained from a capillary puncture, and what implications does this choice have for the accuracy of certain laboratory tests?

A) Arterial blood, which provides the most accurate measure of oxygen saturation for respiratory assessments.

B) Venous blood, which is ideal for testing biochemical markers without the risk of contamination from interstitial fluid.

C) Capillary blood, which is a mixture of arterial and venous blood and can be used for rapid testing but may yield different results compared to venous blood.

D) Whole blood, which is necessary for coagulation studies to ensure accurate results.

83. Capillary tubes are commonly used during capillary punctures to collect blood samples. Which of the following statements best describes their use and significance in laboratory analysis?

A) **To directly inject medication into the bloodstream**—Examine why capillary tubes are not suitable for medication administration and the risks involved in using them for this purpose.

B) **To collect blood samples for laboratory**

analysis—Discuss the advantages of using capillary tubes for sample collection, including their appropriateness for specific tests and situations, and how they facilitate the collection of small blood volumes.

C) **To measure blood pressure**—Evaluate why capillary tubes are not designed for blood pressure measurement and what devices are appropriate for that purpose.

D) **To perform a glucose tolerance test**—Analyze the context in which capillary tubes might be used in glucose testing, but clarify the differences between capillary blood collection and venous blood testing in this procedure.

84. When performing a capillary puncture, the angle at which the puncture is made can impact the success of the procedure. What is the recommended angle for making a capillary puncture?

A) 10-20 degrees

B) 30-45 degrees

C) 45-60 degrees

D) 60-90 degrees

85. Proper disposal of medical waste is essential for maintaining safety and hygiene. How should you dispose of a used lancet after performing a capillary puncture?

A) In the regular trash

B) In a sharps container

C) In a biohazard bag

D) By recycling

86. The accuracy of a capillary puncture test result can be compromised if _____ is applied to the puncture site, as this can cause interstitial fluid to mix with the blood sample.

A) Excessive squeezing

B) Alcohol

C) A sterile lancet

D) Proper identification

87. The microhematocrit tube is commonly used during capillary punctures for specific diagnostic purposes. What is the primary purpose of the microhematocrit tube?

A) To measure blood glucose levels

B) To determine the blood's pH level

C) To assess the percentage of red blood cells in the blood sample

D) To collect plasma for coagulation studies

88. When performing a capillary puncture, it is essential to ensure that the puncture site is free of contamination to avoid compromising test results. What is the best method to ensure that the puncture site is free of contamination?

A) Wipe the site with a dry gauze

B) Use an antiseptic wipe and allow it to dry completely

C) Clean the site with soap and water

D) Apply a bandage to the site after puncture

Cardiovascular System

89. Which of the following blood vessels carries deoxygenated blood from the body back to the heart?

A) Aorta

B) Pulmonary vein

C) Vena cava

D) Carotid artery

90. What is the role of the sinoatrial (SA) node in the heart?

A) To pump blood into the ventricles

B) To generate electrical impulses that initiate the heart's contraction

C) To prevent backflow of blood into the atria

D) To control blood pressure

91. A 60-year-old male patient presents with symptoms of intermittent claudication during physical activity. Upon examination, the healthcare provider notes diminished pulses in the lower extremities. Which of the following statements regarding the characteristics and functions of arteries is most relevant to this patient's condition?

A) Arteries primarily facilitate the exchange of nutrients and waste products with tissues.

B) The thick muscular walls of arteries allow for regulation of blood flow and pressure.

C) All arteries carry oxygenated blood to the body tissues, regardless of their location.

D) Arteries have a larger lumen than veins to accommodate high-volume blood flow.

92. A 55-year-old patient presents with signs of heart failure and has a history of chronic obstructive pulmonary disease (COPD). To assess the patient's cardiovascular function, the healthcare provider reviews the pathway of blood

flow through the heart and lungs. Which of the following sequences accurately represents this pathway, considering the physiological implications of potential obstruction or impairment at each stage?

A) Right atrium → Right ventricle → Pulmonary artery → Lungs → Left atrium → Left ventricle → Aorta

B) Left atrium → Left ventricle → Aorta → Lungs → Right atrium → Right ventricle → Pulmonary artery

C) Right ventricle → Right atrium → Aorta → Lungs → Left ventricle → Left atrium → Pulmonary vein

D) Left ventricle → Aorta → Body → Right atrium → Right ventricle → Pulmonary artery → Lungs

93. The "lub-dub" sounds of the heart are critical indicators of cardiac function during auscultation. Which of the following accurately describes the physiological mechanisms behind these heart sounds?

A) "Lub" is caused by the closure of the aortic and pulmonary valves, while "dub" is caused by the closure of the atrioventricular valves.

B) "Lub" is produced by the closure of the atrioventricular (AV) valves, and "dub" is produced by the closure of the semilunar valves.

C) "Lub" corresponds to ventricular contraction, while "dub" corresponds to atrial contraction.

D) "Lub" is associated with blood flow through the pulmonary veins, and "dub" is associated with blood flow through the aorta.

94. During a clinical assessment, a 72-year-old male patient presents with hypertension and a history of cardiovascular disease. The healthcare provider is reviewing the patient's cardiovascular anatomy and function. Which of the following statements correctly identifies the largest artery in the body and describes its significance in the circulatory system?

A) The pulmonary artery is the largest artery, responsible for carrying oxygenated blood from the lungs to the heart.

B) The aorta is the largest artery, originating from the left ventricle and distributing oxygenated blood to the body.

C) The femoral artery is the largest artery, primarily supplying blood to the lower extremities.

D) The coronary arteries are the largest arteries, as they supply blood directly to the heart muscle.

95. During an EKG analysis, a healthcare professional is evaluating the cardiac cycle of a patient. Which of the following components of the EKG tracing specifically represents the depolarization of the ventricles, and what is its significance in the cardiac cycle?

A) P wave

B) QRS complex

C) T wave

D) U wave

96. A healthcare provider is explaining the role of major veins in the circulatory system to a medical

assistant student. What is the primary function of the superior vena cava, and how does it contribute to overall cardiovascular physiology?

A) To transport oxygenated blood from the lungs to the heart.

B) To carry deoxygenated blood from the lower body to the heart.

C) To return deoxygenated blood from the upper body to the right atrium of the heart.

D) To distribute oxygen-rich blood from the heart to the systemic circulation.

97. During a cardiac physiology lecture, a student asks about the specific function of the atrioventricular (AV) node within the heart's conduction system. Which of the following statements best describes the role of the AV node?

A) The AV node generates electrical impulses that initiate ventricular contraction.

B) The AV node serves as a delay point for electrical impulses, allowing for coordinated contraction of the atria and ventricles.

C) The AV node is responsible for transmitting impulses directly to the atrial myocardium.

D) The AV node facilitates the synchronization of the heart's contractions with the respiratory cycle.

98. In a clinical discussion about heart anatomy and function, a healthcare provider is explaining the role of various structures within the heart. What is the primary purpose of the chordae tendineae, and how do they contribute to proper heart function?

A) To connect the atrioventricular valves to the heart muscle, allowing for direct contraction.

B) To prevent the atrioventricular valves from inverting during ventricular contraction.

C) To facilitate blood flow from the atria to the ventricles during diastole.

D) To anchor the semilunar valves in place during systole.

99. A healthcare provider is reviewing an EKG tracing during a cardiac assessment. What physiological process does the T wave on the EKG represent, and why is it significant in evaluating cardiac health?

A) Atrial depolarization, marking the beginning of atrial contraction.

B) Ventricular depolarization, leading to ventricular contraction.

C) Ventricular repolarization, indicating the recovery phase of the ventricles after contraction.

D) The resting phase of the heart, reflecting the time between beats.

100. During a cardiac assessment, a healthcare provider explains the phases of the cardiac cycle to a student. Which of the following accurately describes a key event that occurs during diastole?

A) The ventricles contract and pump blood into the aorta and pulmonary artery.

B) The atrioventricular (AV) valves close to prevent backflow into the atria.

C) The heart muscle relaxes, and the chambers fill with blood from the atria.

D) The sinoatrial (SA) node fires, initiating a new heartbeat.

101. In a clinical setting, understanding the function of the left atrium is crucial for assessing cardiovascular health. Which of the following scenarios best demonstrates the physiological role of the left atrium in the cardiac cycle, particularly in relation to maintaining effective hemodynamics?

A) During atrial fibrillation, the left atrium experiences ineffective contractions, leading to stasis of blood and an increased risk of thrombus formation.

B) Following pulmonary surgery, the left atrium compensates for reduced blood flow by increasing its volume capacity, allowing for greater reservoir function.

C) In cases of mitral valve stenosis, the left atrium becomes dilated due to increased pressure from the left ventricle, indicating compromised blood flow to the systemic circulation.

D) During physical exertion, the left atrium enhances its contractility to push more blood into the left ventricle, thereby improving cardiac output during exercise.

102. In a clinical scenario, a healthcare provider is explaining the importance of understanding ventricular systole in relation to overall heart function and patient health. Which of the following statements most accurately reflects the physiological events of ventricular systole and suggests why these events are critical for maintaining cardiovascular health?

A) Ventricular systole initiates with the opening of the atrioventricular (AV) valves, which allows for maximum filling of the ventricles, ensuring adequate stroke volume during the next heartbeat.

B) During ventricular systole, the ventricles contract vigorously, resulting in increased intraventricular pressure that closes the AV valves and ejects blood into the systemic and pulmonary circulation, which is vital for delivering oxygen and nutrients to tissues.

C) This phase involves a prolonged relaxation of the heart muscle, enabling the ventricles to refill completely with blood from the atria, which is essential for optimal cardiac output during physical activity.

D) Ventricular systole is marked by the firing of the sinoatrial (SA) node, triggering a series of electrical impulses that lead to the contraction of the atria and ventricles in unison, promoting efficient blood flow throughout the heart.

103. A patient presents with symptoms of tissue hypoxia and fatigue. After examining the patient's medical history, you suspect a possible issue with capillary function. Which of the following statements best describes how impaired capillary exchange might contribute to the patient's condition?

A) Impaired capillary exchange would lead to an increase in blood pressure, which directly causes tissue hypoxia due to inadequate perfusion.

B) Dysfunctional capillaries may hinder the diffusion of oxygen from the blood into the tissues, resulting in decreased oxygen availability and subsequent fatigue.

C) If capillaries are compromised, waste products will accumulate in the blood, leading to systemic toxicity rather than localized tissue hypoxia.

D) Capillaries play a minimal role in nutrient and gas exchange; therefore, impaired exchange would not significantly affect tissue oxygenation.

Hemostasis and the Coagulation

104. A patient is diagnosed with a bleeding disorder characterized by prolonged aPTT (activated partial thromboplastin time). Considering the role of various clotting factors, which of the following factors is most critical to the proper functioning of the intrinsic pathway of

coagulation, and what implication does its deficiency have on hemostasis?

A) Factor VII; its deficiency primarily affects the extrinsic pathway, leading to a minor increase in bleeding risk.

B) Factor XII; its deficiency results in significant bleeding due to impaired initial activation of the intrinsic pathway.

C) Factor IX; its deficiency can cause hemophilia B, resulting in severe bleeding episodes despite normal levels of other factors.

D) Factor I; its deficiency leads to failure of fibrin formation, affecting both intrinsic and extrinsic pathways significantly.

105. In the context of hemostasis and the management of coagulation disorders, which vitamin plays a pivotal role in the synthesis of clotting factors in the liver, and how does its deficiency impact coagulation?

A) Vitamin A

B) Vitamin C

C) Vitamin K

D) Vitamin D

106. A clinician is interpreting a patient's D-dimer test results as part of a workup for suspected thrombosis. Considering the physiological processes involved in coagulation and fibrinolysis, what is the primary significance of elevated D-dimer levels in this context, and how should the results influence the management plan?

A) Elevated D-dimer levels indicate a deficiency in clotting factors, necessitating replacement therapy to prevent bleeding complications.

B) Elevated D-dimer levels suggest active clot formation and breakdown, prompting further investigation for conditions like deep vein thrombosis (DVT) or pulmonary embolism (PE).

C) Elevated D-dimer levels reflect a failure of platelet aggregation, indicating that platelet function tests should be performed to evaluate hemostasis.

D) Elevated D-dimer levels are irrelevant in the

context of thrombotic disorders and should be disregarded in clinical decision-making.

107. A patient with a history of atrial fibrillation is prescribed warfarin to prevent thromboembolic events. Considering the pharmacological action of warfarin, what is the primary mechanism by which this anticoagulant exerts its effects, and what important considerations should be made regarding its use?

A) Warfarin inhibits platelet aggregation by blocking the action of thromboxane A2, reducing the risk of arterial clots.

B) Warfarin directly inhibits thrombin, leading to a decrease in fibrin formation and stabilization of clots.

C) Warfarin inhibits vitamin K-dependent clotting factors, reducing the synthesis of factors II, VII, IX, and X, which requires regular monitoring of INR for dosage adjustments.

D) Warfarin enhances the activity of tissue factor,

promoting rapid clot formation in response to vascular injury.

108. During the hemostasis process, platelets are primarily responsible for _____, which involves adhering to the site of injury and releasing signals that initiate the coagulation cascade.

A) Carrying oxygen to tissues

B) Forming a platelet plug

C) Producing antibodies

D) Breaking down blood clots

109. The platelet aggregation test is used to assess platelet function by measuring how well platelets clump together in response to various agonists.

A) True
B) False

110. The conversion of prothrombin to thrombin is a critical step in the coagulation cascade. In which phase does this conversion occur, and what are the implications for hemostasis and clot formation?

A) **Primary hemostasis**—Discuss why this phase, involving platelet adhesion and aggregation, does not include the conversion of prothrombin, and the significance of this process in initial wound response.

B) **Secondary hemostasis**—Analyze how the conversion of prothrombin to thrombin signifies a shift from primary to secondary hemostasis, detailing the cascade of reactions that lead to clot stabilization and the role of thrombin in activating additional clotting factors.

C) **Fibrinolysis**—Evaluate the role of fibrinolysis in the coagulation process and why it occurs after clot formation, contrasting it with the active formation of thrombin.

D) **Platelet aggregation**—Examine the role of thrombin in promoting platelet aggregation and how its production is essential for effective clot formation, while clarifying the distinction between thrombin production and platelet function.

111. In the complex cascade of the coagulation process, thrombin plays a pivotal role. What is the primary function of thrombin, and how does its activity impact both clot formation and the overall hemostatic response?

A) Thrombin initiates the coagulation cascade by activating vitamin K-dependent clotting factors, enhancing the overall clotting response.

B) Thrombin functions as an anticoagulant, preventing excessive clot formation and promoting fibrinolysis to maintain blood flow.

C) Thrombin converts fibrinogen to fibrin and activates platelets, thereby amplifying the coagulation cascade and promoting stable clot formation.

D) Thrombin serves to dissolve existing clots by breaking down fibrin, thus preventing the obstruction of blood vessels.

112. The condition known as _____ is associated with an increased risk of excessive bleeding due to a deficiency in specific clotting factors, which impairs the body's ability to form stable blood clots.

A) Thrombocytopenia

B) Hemophilia

C) Leukemia

D) Polycythemia vera

113. Calcium ions (Ca^{2+}) are essential in the coagulation process, influencing several steps in the hemostatic cascade. Which statement best describes the critical role of calcium ions in coagulation, and what are the implications for clot formation and stability?

A) They activate platelets for aggregation

B) They stabilize the fibrin clot

C) They facilitate the conversion of prothrombin to thrombin

D) They initiate fibrinolysis

114. A healthcare provider is evaluating a patient with a suspected bleeding disorder. The patient's laboratory results show a significantly prolonged activated partial thromboplastin time (aPTT). Which of the following interpretations regarding the aPTT and its clinical implications is most accurate?

A) A prolonged aPTT suggests a deficiency in the extrinsic pathway, specifically involving Factor VII, indicating a high risk for venous thrombosis.

B) Prolongation of aPTT primarily indicates a deficiency in the intrinsic pathway or the common pathway, possibly due to deficiencies in Factors VIII, IX, XI, or XII, which may lead to hemophilia-like symptoms.

C) The aPTT test is primarily used to assess the overall clotting capability of the blood, regardless of which pathway is affected, and does not specify intrinsic or extrinsic issues.

D) A prolonged aPTT is typically an indication of

platelet dysfunction rather than a deficiency in coagulation factors, suggesting a need for platelet aggregation studies.

115. A 45-year-old patient presents with a deep laceration resulting from a fall. Upon assessment, you understand that the body's hemostatic response involves the activation of various coagulation pathways. Which of the following statements correctly describes the role of the intrinsic pathway of coagulation in response to endothelial injury?

A) The intrinsic pathway is primarily activated by tissue factor released from damaged tissues and is critical for initial platelet aggregation.

B) Endothelial injury exposes collagen, which activates Factor XII, leading to a cascade of reactions involving factors XI, IX, and VIII, ultimately forming a fibrin clot.

C) The intrinsic pathway operates independently of the common pathway and does not contribute to the final clot formation in hemostasis.

D) Activation of the intrinsic pathway leads to a direct increase in platelet production from the bone marrow in response to vascular damage.

116. A patient presents with recurrent deep vein thrombosis (DVT) and a family history of similar events. Considering the clinical characteristics and underlying mechanisms of various clotting disorders, which condition is most likely associated with an excessive tendency to form clots in the blood vessels?

A) Hemophilia

B) Thrombophilia

C) Disseminated intravascular coagulation (DIC)

D) Von Willebrand disease

117. In the context of coagulation testing, which anticoagulant is commonly utilized in blood collection tubes, and what is its mechanism of

action regarding calcium ions in the coagulation cascade?

A) Sodium citrate

B) Heparin

C) EDTA

D) Warfarin

118. The protein _____ is NOT involved in the coagulation cascade, as it primarily functions in the transportation of oxygen in red blood cells.

A) Factor VII

B) Fibrinogen

C) Thrombin

D) Hemoglobin

Laboratory Operations

119 A laboratory technician is preparing to analyze a blood sample. They will use a centrifuge as part of the sample processing. What is the primary function of the centrifuge in this context, and why is it critical for subsequent analyses?

A) The centrifuge mixes the blood sample thoroughly, ensuring that all components are uniformly distributed for accurate testing.

B) The centrifuge separates the blood components based on their density, allowing for the isolation of plasma and cellular elements necessary for various tests.

C) The centrifuge sterilizes the blood sample, eliminating any potential contaminants before further analysis.

D) The centrifuge regulates the temperature of the blood sample during processing, preserving the integrity of temperature-sensitive components.

120. The main purpose of a hemoglobin A1c (HbA1c) test in a laboratory is to _____,

providing insight into long-term blood glucose control for diabetic patients.

A) Diagnose anemia

B) Monitor long-term blood glucose control

C) Assess liver function

D) Measure blood oxygen levels

121. Which of the following best describes the proper procedure for performing a venipuncture?

A. Insert the needle at a 45-degree angle and draw blood slowly

B. Insert the needle at a 15-30 degree angle and draw blood quickly

C. Insert the needle parallel to the vein and draw blood at a moderate pace

D. Insert the needle perpendicular to the vein and draw blood slowly

122. Which of the following is an important factor in ensuring the quality of blood specimens?

A. Using the same needle for multiple draws

B. Filling tubes to the specified level

C. Shaking the tubes vigorously

D. Allowing the sample to sit at room temperature for several days

123. What type of specimen is typically collected for a culture and sensitivity test?

A. Serum

B. Urine

C. Plasma

D. Whole blood

124. Sodium citrate is the commonly used additive in blood collection tubes for coagulation tests because it effectively prevents blood clotting by binding calcium ions, which are necessary for the clotting process.

A) True

B) False

125. Following the CLSI guidelines for blood collection, the order of draw starts with the light blue top tube for coagulation tests, followed by the red top tube, and concludes with the gray top tube for glucose testing.

A) True

B) False

126. In the context of laboratory diagnostics, which test is predominantly performed using a serum sample, and what factors contribute to its preference over other sample types?

A) Complete blood count (CBC)

B) Basic metabolic panel (BMP)

C) Coagulation studies (PT/aPTT)

D) Urinalysis

127. The term _____ is used to describe an abnormally low platelet count, which can lead to an increased risk of bleeding and bruising.

A) Thrombocytosis

B) Thrombocytopenia

C) Hemophilia

D) Leukopenia

128. The term "hematoma" refers to which of the following?

A) A benign tumor of blood vessels.

B) A localized collection of blood outside of blood vessels, typically due to injury or trauma.

C) A condition characterized by low platelet count leading to excessive bleeding.

D) A procedure for drawing blood samples from a vein.

129. Polycythemia is a condition that involves an abnormal increase in red blood cells. Which of the following best explains the potential causes and complications associated with polycythemia?

A) Polycythemia is primarily caused by a deficiency in red blood cell production, leading to anemia-related complications.

B) Polycythemia occurs when there is an abnormal increase in red blood cells, which can thicken the blood and increase the risk of complications like clots, strokes, or heart attacks.

C) Polycythemia results from an excess number of white blood cells and is most commonly linked to infections or autoimmune disorders.

D) Polycythemia is characterized by an elevated platelet count, leading to excessive bleeding or clotting disorders.

130. A 58-year-old patient with a history of hypertension and hyperlipidemia presents with leg pain during walking and reduced pulses in the lower extremities. Imaging reveals narrowed

arteries with calcified walls. Based on the patient's presentation and imaging, which of the following best describes the pathophysiology of arteriosclerosis, and what are the potential consequences if left untreated?

A) Arteriosclerosis is caused by inflammation of the arterial walls, leading to the immediate rupture of arteries and severe bleeding, particularly in the extremities.

B) Arteriosclerosis results in the thickening and hardening of the arterial walls due to calcium deposition, reduced elasticity, and narrowed vessel lumen, increasing the risk of ischemia and tissue necrosis.

C) Arteriosclerosis is a reversible condition characterized by plaque buildup in the venous system, which can be completely treated through lifestyle changes and cholesterol-lowering medications.

D) Arteriosclerosis leads to vasodilation and increased blood flow, resulting in symptoms such as severe hypotension, but it does not increase the risk of cardiovascular events.

131. In medical terminology, the suffix "-cytosis" is used to describe certain conditions related to cell counts. Which of the following best explains the significance of "-cytosis" in a clinical context, and what might be the physiological or pathological implications of this finding?

A) **Enlargement of cells**—Examine the potential for "-cytosis" to reflect changes in cell size, clarifying the difference between increased cell number and cell enlargement (e.g., -megaly) in diagnostic contexts.

B) **Decrease in cell count**—Analyze why "-cytosis" does not indicate a decrease in cell numbers and explore the alternative terminology for reduced cell counts (e.g., -penia) and its clinical significance.

C) **Increase in cell count**—Discuss how "-cytosis" indicates an increase in the number of specific cell types, including possible causes such as infection, inflammation, or malignancy, and explain how this affects diagnostic and therapeutic decisions.

D) **Death of cells**—Consider why "-cytosis" does not refer to cell death and explain the appropriate terms (e.g., necrosis or apoptosis) that are used to describe cell death in pathological states.

132. The term "phlebotomy" has historical and clinical significance in medicine. Which of the following best describes the literal meaning of the term and its application in modern healthcare?

A) **Cutting into an artery**—Discuss why this description is incorrect for phlebotomy and clarify the specific medical procedures that involve arteries.

B) **Incision into a vein**—Analyze the literal meaning of phlebotomy, focusing on its historical roots in vein incision and how it has evolved into a less invasive procedure using needles in modern medical practice.

C) **Removal of blood**—Evaluate how the process of phlebotomy often involves blood removal, but emphasize why this is a secondary outcome rather than the literal meaning of the term.

D) **Puncturing the skin**—Examine why skin puncture is a part of modern phlebotomy, but not its primary definition, and differentiate this from other procedures like skin biopsies or injections.

133. The suffix "-penia" is commonly encountered in clinical diagnoses, indicating specific physiological deficiencies. Which of the following best explains the significance of "-penia" in medical terminology, and what are the potential clinical consequences of such a condition?

A) Increase in cell count

B) Decrease in cell count

C) Destruction of cells

D) Formation of cells

134. A 65-year-old patient develops deep vein thrombosis (DVT) and is placed on anticoagulation therapy. The attending physician explains that the body's natural mechanism will eventually break down the blood clot. Which of

the following terms refers to the physiological process of blood clot breakdown, and what key enzyme is involved in this process?

A) Thrombopoiesis

B) Fibrinolysis

C) Hemostasis

D) Coagulation

135. Understanding the prefixes used in medical terminology can provide insight into anatomical structures and clinical procedures. Which of the following prefixes specifically refers to "vein," and how does its application differ from other related terms in the vascular system?

A) **Hemo-**—Discuss why this prefix refers to blood itself rather than the specific structures (such as veins or arteries) that carry blood.

B) **Veno-**—Examine how this prefix also refers to veins and compare its usage in clinical practice with "phlebo-" in terms such as venography versus phlebotomy.

C) **Phlebo-**—Analyze how this prefix refers specifically to veins, as seen in terms like phlebotomy or phlebitis, and discuss its relevance in diagnostic and therapeutic procedures involving the venous system.

D) **Angio-**—Evaluate why this prefix refers to vessels in general (both veins and arteries) and how it applies in broader vascular contexts like angioplasty or angiogenesis.

Specimen Collection and Handling

136. **A phlebotomist is preparing to draw blood from a patient and applies a tourniquet to the upper arm. Which of the following best explains the recommended time limit for tourniquet application, and what could happen if the tourniquet is left in place for longer than the recommended duration?**

A) The tourniquet should be applied for no more than 3 minutes; prolonged application can increase blood pressure and may cause vascular collapse.

B) The tourniquet should be applied for no longer than 1 minute; prolonged application may lead to hemoconcentration and inaccurate test results due to falsely elevated levels of blood components.

C) The tourniquet can remain in place for up to 5 minutes; this maximizes the visibility of veins without impacting the quality of the blood sample.

D) There is no time limit for tourniquet application during venipuncture, as it only affects the surface veins and not the integrity of the blood sample.

137. When performing venipuncture in the antecubital space, selecting the proper needle angle is critical for successful blood collection. What is the recommended needle insertion angle, and how does this angle impact the procedure?

A) 5-10 degrees, as a shallow angle helps minimize patient discomfort and prevents the needle from passing through the vein wall.

B) 15-30 degrees, allowing the needle to enter the vein smoothly without puncturing through it, while also ensuring that the bevel is fully within the vein lumen for optimal blood flow.

C) 45-60 degrees, as this angle provides better control over the needle and ensures that it can penetrate deeper veins located in the antecubital space.

D) 75-90 degrees, used when veins are particularly difficult to access and when a deeper needle insertion is necessary for blood flow.

138. In laboratory diagnostics, choosing the correct blood collection tube is essential for ensuring accurate test results, especially for coagulation studies. Which of the following blood collection tubes is the most appropriate for coagulation tests, and why is the anticoagulant in this tube particularly suited for such studies?

A) Red top (no additives)

B) Lavender top (EDTA)

C) Light blue top (sodium citrate)

D) Green top (heparin)

139. A phlebotomist collects a blood sample from a patient for a series of diagnostic tests. To prevent mislabeling errors and ensure the integrity of the sample, what is the most appropriate method for labeling the specimen, and why is this step critical to patient safety?

A) The specimen should be labeled prior to collection with pre-printed labels, ensuring efficient workflow and faster turnaround times.

B) The specimen should be labeled immediately after collection and while still in the presence of the patient, ensuring proper patient identification and preventing mix-ups.

C) Specimens can be labeled anytime after collection, as long as they are stored correctly to prevent contamination.

D) It is sufficient to label specimens before sending them to the lab, as this reduces interruptions during patient care and minimizes the risk of mislabeling.

140. Blood specimens must meet certain criteria to be accepted for laboratory testing. Which of the following scenarios would warrant specimen rejection by the laboratory, and why is proper collection and labeling crucial for accurate diagnostic results?

A) The specimen was collected in the correct tube, but there is minor hemolysis. This is acceptable as long as the hemolysis does not affect critical analytes.

B) The specimen tube is expired, or the blood has clotted in a tube meant for anticoagulation testing, which compromises test accuracy and leads to rejection.

C) The specimen is labeled properly, but the blood was drawn from the wrong anatomical site, making it more prone to rejection.

D) The specimen is slightly underfilled, but within the acceptable range for testing, so it should still be processed without issue.

141. During a venipuncture procedure, the phlebotomist aims to collect a high-quality blood sample without causing hemolysis. Which of the following practices is most effective for minimizing the risk of hemolysis, and why is this important for ensuring accurate laboratory results?

A) Using a smaller needle (25-gauge) and rapidly injecting blood into the collection tube, ensuring fast sample processing.

B) Using a large-bore needle (18-gauge) and vigorously shaking the tube to ensure proper mixing of anticoagulants with the blood.

C) Using the correct needle size (21-23 gauge), allowing blood to flow gently into the collection tube, and gently inverting the tube after collection to mix the blood with anticoagulants.

D) Using a syringe to draw blood, then forcefully injecting the blood into the tube, preventing clots from forming in the sample.

142. A phlebotomist is preparing to perform venipuncture on a pediatric patient with small veins. Which of the following needle sizes is most appropriate for minimizing discomfort and preventing vein damage, and why is this selection critical for ensuring a successful blood draw?

A) 18-gauge; this needle size ensures fast blood flow, reducing the overall time of the procedure.

B) 21-gauge; this needle size is the standard for most adults but may still be too large for smaller veins.

C) 23-gauge; this needle size is thin enough to minimize vein damage and prevent collapse while still allowing sufficient blood flow.

D) 25-gauge; this very small needle size completely eliminates discomfort and allows a rapid blood draw.

143. When performing venipuncture on a patient with an IV in one arm, the blood should ideally be drawn from the arm without the IV. If this is not possible, the venipuncture should be performed below the IV site after stopping the IV to avoid contamination.

A) True

B) False

144. A phlebotomist is preparing to perform a capillary blood collection on an adult patient for a point-of-care test. Which of the following sites is most appropriate for obtaining the blood sample, and why is this site preferred over other locations?

A) The center of the fingertip on the index finger, as it has a higher concentration of capillaries for better blood flow.

B) The side of the fingertip on the ring or middle finger, to minimize discomfort and access an area with good capillary flow.

C) The earlobe, as it ensures more rapid blood flow without the risk of damaging nerve endings.

D) The palm of the hand, as it avoids sensitive nerve endings found in the fingers and provides a flat surface for collection.

145. A patient with a history of a left-sided mastectomy presents for a routine blood draw. Which of the following practices should the healthcare provider follow when choosing a venipuncture site, and why is this protocol critical for patient safety?

A) Draw blood from the left arm, but use a smaller needle to minimize the risk of complications.

B) Perform the blood draw on the opposite arm (right arm), as the left arm may have impaired lymphatic drainage and increased risk of lymphedema.

C) Use the left arm for venipuncture, but avoid using a tourniquet to prevent additional pressure on the lymphatic system.

D) Blood can be drawn from either arm as long as proper aseptic technique is followed to prevent infection.

146. A potential complication of performing a heel stick in infants is _____, which can

occur if the puncture is too deep and reaches the bone.

A) Nerve damage

B) Osteomyelitis (bone infection)

C) Hemolysis

D) Hematoma

147. Leaving a tourniquet on for longer than one minute during venipuncture can result in hemoconcentration, which may lead to inaccurate laboratory results by increasing the concentration of blood cells and solutes. It can also cause patient discomfort and increase the risk of bruising.

A) True
B) False

148. A phlebotomist is about to perform a venipuncture on a patient who has an active IV line in the left arm. Which of the following actions is the best approach to avoid contamination of the

blood sample, and why is this precaution essential for accurate lab results?

A) Draw blood from the same arm but above the IV insertion site to avoid interference from the IV fluids.

B) Perform the venipuncture from the same arm as the IV line but use a larger needle to ensure a pure blood sample.

C) Draw blood from the opposite arm if possible, or below the IV insertion site if an alternate site is unavailable, to prevent dilution or contamination of the sample.

D) Turn off the IV line for 2 minutes and then draw the blood from the same site where the IV is located.

149. When handling blood collection tubes containing anticoagulants, it is essential to use the correct inversion technique to ensure proper mixing. Which of the following best describes the procedure for inverting these tubes, and why is this technique critical for accurate test results?

A) Invert the tube vigorously 20 times to rapidly mix the blood and anticoagulant, ensuring quick anticoagulation and preventing clotting.

B) Invert the tube slowly once, then let it sit upright to allow natural mixing of the anticoagulant with the blood.

C) Invert the tube gently 5-10 times immediately after collection, as this prevents clot formation and avoids hemolysis while ensuring thorough mixing of the blood and anticoagulant.

D) Leave the tube undisturbed for 30 minutes to allow the anticoagulant to naturally bind with the blood cells, reducing the risk of hemolysis.

150. A phlebotomist is preparing to collect a blood sample from a patient who is dehydrated and has difficult-to-locate veins. Which method would be most effective for ensuring a successful blood draw, and what additional techniques can be used to enhance vein visibility and accessibility?

A) Use a standard straight needle and draw blood from the forearm to access larger veins.

B) Use a butterfly needle and apply warm compresses to the arm to help dilate the veins before the draw.

C) Perform a fingerstick instead of venipuncture, as it is less invasive and provides sufficient blood for most tests.

D) Draw blood quickly with a larger gauge needle to minimize the time the vein is under pressure.

Venipuncture Techniques

151. The timing of releasing the tourniquet during venipuncture is critical for both patient safety and the accuracy of blood test results. Which of the following best explains why the tourniquet must be released before the needle is withdrawn, and how this impacts blood collection?

A) Releasing the tourniquet after withdrawing the needle is recommended to prevent backflow of blood into the vein, minimizing the risk of post-puncture bleeding.

B) The tourniquet should remain in place until the needle is withdrawn to maintain vein visibility and ensure consistent blood flow into the collection tube.

C) Releasing the tourniquet before withdrawing the needle prevents **hemoconcentration**, which can affect analyte concentrations and lead to inaccurate test results, while also reducing the risk of hematoma formation.

D) The tourniquet should only be released if the vein collapses during the procedure, to ensure continued blood flow for the remainder of the venipuncture.

152. A key indicator that the needle has entered the vein properly during venipuncture is the _____, confirming that the vein has been accessed correctly.

A) Patient experiencing pain at the puncture site

B) Sudden appearance of blood in the hub of the needle

C) Needle meeting resistance upon insertion

D) Tourniquet becoming loose

153. For optimal comfort and accuracy during venipuncture, the patient should be seated comfortably with their arm supported on a flat surface, or lying down if there is a risk of fainting.

A) True
B) False

154. The use of a tourniquet is a critical component of the venipuncture process. Which of the following statements best describes the primary purpose of a tourniquet during this procedure, and what are the potential implications of improper use?

A) **To sterilize the skin**—Evaluate why the primary function of a tourniquet is not related to skin antisepsis, and discuss the appropriate methods for preparing the skin prior to venipuncture.

B) **To constrict blood flow and make veins more visible**—Analyze how this technique enhances vein prominence and why it is essential for successful venipuncture, considering factors such as vein anatomy and patient variability.

C) **To minimize patient discomfort**—Discuss the role of the tourniquet in patient comfort, examining how effective vein selection and technique contribute more significantly to minimizing discomfort during the procedure.

D) **To prevent hematoma formation**—Examine the relationship between tourniquet use and hematoma risk, discussing how improper application and prolonged use can actually increase the likelihood of hematoma development.

155. What is the correct procedure if a blood sample needs to be collected for both coagulation studies and serum chemistry tests?

A) Collect the coagulation sample first, then the serum sample

B) Collect the serum sample first, then the coagulation sample

C) Collect both samples simultaneously using different needles

D) Use the same tube for both types of tests

156. One of the most common causes of hemolysis in blood samples is the use of a needle that is too small, which can cause red blood cells to rupture during collection, leading to inaccurate test results.

A) True

B) False

157. A phlebotomist prepares to perform venipuncture on a patient. What is the primary purpose of applying a tourniquet, and what considerations should be taken into account to ensure optimal results during the blood draw?

A) To prevent arterial blood flow, ensuring that only venous blood is collected for accurate testing.

B) To engorge the veins, making them more visible and easier to puncture for blood collection.

C) To minimize patient discomfort by restricting blood flow and reducing vein movement during the draw.

D) To increase the pressure in the veins, facilitating a faster blood draw with less time spent at the site.

158. The primary purpose of using a capillary tube for blood collection is to _____, often for diagnostic testing such as glucose levels or hematocrit.

A) Collect large volumes of blood for transfusion

B) Obtain small blood samples for testing

C) Assess oxygen levels in arterial blood

D) Store blood for long-term use

159. When collecting blood using a syringe, specific techniques are vital to minimize the risk of hemolysis. Which of the following methods is most effective in preventing hemolysis, and why is

this technique important for ensuring sample integrity?

A) Pulling back the plunger rapidly to create a vacuum effect helps fill the syringe quickly and is sufficient to avoid hemolysis.

B) Using a larger bore needle allows for faster blood flow, reducing the risk of hemolysis by minimizing friction and turbulence.

C) Inserting the needle at a steep angle ensures optimal access to the vein, but pulling back the plunger quickly may lead to hemolysis.

D) Gently pulling back the plunger slowly reduces turbulence during collection, minimizing shear forces on red blood cells and thereby preventing hemolysis.

160. A phlebotomist is assessing the best approach for drawing blood from a patient with small, fragile veins and a history of difficulty during venipuncture. In which of the following scenarios would using a winged infusion set (butterfly needle) be the most appropriate choice?

A) The patient is a healthy adult with easily visible veins, requiring a routine blood draw for a comprehensive metabolic panel.

B) The patient is a pediatric patient with small veins, and the phlebotomist anticipates a need for precise control during the blood collection.

C) The patient requires a large volume of blood for testing, necessitating the use of a standard needle to ensure an adequate sample.

D) The patient is undergoing a blood transfusion, and a standard needle is required for faster blood flow.

ANSWERS WITH EXPLANATION

Anatomy and Physiology

1. Answer: B) Median cubital vein

Explanation: The median cubital vein is the most appropriate vein for venipuncture because it is centrally located, superficial, and easily accessible, reducing the risk of hitting nearby arteries or nerves. It is also relatively stable during venipuncture, making it less likely to roll or cause discomfort to the patient. While the basilic and cephalic veins can be used, the basilic vein is located near the brachial artery and nerves, which increases the risk of complications. The cephalic vein is often more difficult to palpate and may be uncomfortable for the patient. The femoral vein is used in more critical situations and is not a standard site for routine blood draws.

2. Answer: C) To transport oxygen from the lungs to tissues and carry carbon dioxide back to the lungs

Explanation: Erythrocytes, commonly known as red blood cells, are specialized for gas transport. Their primary function is to carry oxygen from the lungs to all the tissues in the body, which is essential for cellular respiration and energy production.

Hemoglobin within erythrocytes binds to oxygen in the lungs and releases it in tissues that need it. Additionally, erythrocytes help remove carbon dioxide, a waste product of metabolism, by transporting it back to the lungs, where it is exhaled.

3. Answer: B) Urinary system, through renal mechanisms that control the excretion of hydrogen ions (H+) and the reabsorption of bicarbonate (HCO3-)

Explanation: The **urinary system**, specifically the kidneys, provides long-term regulation of blood pH by adjusting the concentration of hydrogen ions and reabsorbing bicarbonate ions. When the body's pH is too acidic, the kidneys excrete more hydrogen ions in the urine and reabsorb more bicarbonate into the bloodstream. Conversely, when the pH is too alkaline, the kidneys decrease hydrogen ion excretion and reduce bicarbonate reabsorption.

4. Answer: B) Myocardium

Explanation: The myocardium, the thick middle layer of the heart, is made of specialized cardiac muscle cells that contract to pump blood throughout the body. When the myocardium is weakened or damaged, such as in heart failure, the heart's ability to generate sufficient force to pump blood effectively is reduced. This leads to inadequate circulation of oxygen and nutrients, causing symptoms like fatigue, shortness of breath, and fluid retention due to the heart's reduced efficiency. The endocardium, epicardium, and pericardium serve other functions, such as lining the heart and providing protection, but they do not contribute to the heart's pumping action.

5. Answer: C) Pulmonary vein

Explanation: The pulmonary vein is unique because it is one of the few veins in the body that carries oxygenated blood. It transports oxygen-rich blood from the lungs back to the left atrium of the heart, where it can then be pumped into the left ventricle and out to the rest of the body via the aorta.

6. Answer: C) Alveoli, specialized for efficient gas exchange due to their thin walls and proximity to pulmonary capillaries

Explanation: The **alveoli** are the primary functional units of the lungs where gas exchange occurs. These tiny sac-like structures are surrounded by a dense capillary network and are lined by a single layer of squamous epithelial cells (type I alveolar cells) to minimize the diffusion distance for gases. The extensive surface area provided by millions of alveoli in the lungs allows for a high rate of oxygen and carbon dioxide exchange, which is critical for maintaining efficient respiration and blood gas levels.

7. Answer: C) Platelets, which adhere to the site of vascular injury, release thromboxane, and promote fibrin formation

Explanation: Platelets play a pivotal role in the initiation of hemostasis by adhering to exposed collagen fibers at the site of vessel damage. Upon activation, platelets release several key substances, such as **thromboxane A2**, which enhances platelet aggregation and vasoconstriction, and **serotonin**, which also promotes vasoconstriction. Platelets also release factors that activate the **coagulation cascade**, leading to the conversion of fibrinogen to fibrin—a protein that stabilizes the platelet plug by forming a mesh that traps additional platelets and blood cells, forming a clot.

8. Answer: A) True

Explanation: The motor cortex in the cerebral cortex is crucial for initiating and coordinating voluntary movements. It sends signals to the muscles to execute these movements. In contrast, the spinal cord is involved in reflex actions, which are automatic responses to stimuli that do not require conscious thought.

9. Answer: D) White blood cells (WBCs)

Explanation: White blood cells (leukocytes) are vital in immune defense, recognizing and neutralizing harmful pathogens like bacteria, viruses, and other foreign particles. Unlike red blood cells, which carry oxygen, and platelets, which aid in clotting, WBCs are specifically involved in immunity.

10. Answer: B) False

Explanation: The process of hemostasis includes several key steps: vascular spasm, platelet plug formation, and coagulation. Additionally, it also involves clot retraction, which helps in stabilizing the clot, and fibrinolysis, which is the process of breaking down the clot once the vessel has healed. Thus, the statement is false as it omits these crucial components of hemostasis.

11. Answer: D) Type O

Explanation: Type O negative blood is called the universal donor because it lacks both A and B antigens, as well as the Rh factor, meaning it can be given to patients of any blood type without triggering an immune response. This makes it especially valuable in emergency situations when a patient's blood type is unknown.

12. Answer: C) Returning excess interstitial fluid to the bloodstream

Explanation: The lymphatic system's most critical function in preventing fluid accumulation (edema) is its role in returning excess interstitial fluid that escapes from the blood capillaries back to the bloodstream. When the lymphatic system is impaired, fluid can accumulate in tissues, causing swelling (lymphedema). This occurs because the system fails to adequately drain the lymph, leading to fluid retention in the legs and ankles. While the lymphatic system also plays a role in immune response by producing lymphocytes and fighting infection, its dysfunction primarily results in fluid imbalances rather than impairing oxygen transport or nutrient absorption.

13. Answer: C) To initiate blood clot formation to prevent excessive bleeding

Explanation: The primary function of platelets is to prevent excessive bleeding by forming blood clots. When a blood vessel is injured, platelets adhere to the site, become activated, and release substances that attract more platelets. This aggregation of platelets forms a plug that helps seal the wound. Platelets also work in conjunction with clotting factors in the blood to form a stable clot.

14. Answer: B) Liver, which detoxifies the blood via enzymatic pathways such as cytochrome P450, converting lipophilic toxins into hydrophilic compounds for excretion

Explanation: The **liver** is the primary organ responsible for detoxifying the blood. It utilizes specialized enzymes, most notably the **cytochrome P450 enzyme system**, to metabolize harmful substances. These enzymes perform **phase I reactions** (oxidation, reduction, hydrolysis) to convert lipophilic toxins into more polar metabolites. These metabolites are further processed in **phase II reactions** (conjugation), where they are conjugated with molecules such as glucuronic acid or sulfate, making them water-soluble. This allows the toxins to be excreted in bile or urine.

15. Answer: B) To transport oxygen from the lungs to tissues and carbon dioxide from tissues to the lungs

Explanation: Hemoglobin is the protein in red blood cells responsible for binding oxygen in the lungs and transporting it to tissues throughout the body, where it is released for cellular respiration. Hemoglobin also plays a role in carrying carbon dioxide, a waste product of metabolism, from the tissues back to the lungs for exhalation. This gas exchange is essential for maintaining proper oxygen and carbon dioxide levels in the body.

16. Answer: B) Small intestine

Explanation: The small intestine is primarily responsible for nutrient absorption, with its specialized structure—villi and microvilli—maximizing surface area for effective absorption of carbohydrates, proteins, fats, vitamins, and minerals.

If there is a dysfunction in the small intestine, such as in conditions like celiac disease, Crohn's disease, or infections, the body may not absorb essential nutrients effectively. This can lead to malnutrition, as nutrients are not sufficiently taken up into the bloodstream, resulting in weight loss and deficiencies. The stomach aids in digestion but does not absorb nutrients, the large intestine absorbs water and electrolytes, and the esophagus serves merely as a conduit for food.

17. Answer: B) Insulin

Explanation: Insulin is a hormone produced by the pancreas that helps regulate blood glucose levels by promoting the uptake of glucose into cells, particularly in the liver, muscle, and fat tissue. This process lowers blood glucose levels. Glucagon, also produced by the pancreas, has the opposite effect, raising blood glucose levels by stimulating the release of glucose from the liver. Adrenaline and cortisol are stress hormones that can also influence blood glucose levels, but they do not promote glucose uptake into cells.

18. Answer: C) Sinoatrial (SA) node

Explanation: The sinoatrial (SA) node, located in the upper part of the right atrium, acts as the natural pacemaker of the heart. It produces electrical signals that initiate each heartbeat, setting the pace for the heart's contractions. This impulse then travels through the atria and ventricles, ensuring the heart pumps blood efficiently.

19. Answer: B) False

Explanation: The primary function of the large intestine is to absorb water and electrolytes from indigestible food residues and to form and store feces. While it does play a role in the fermentation of some materials by gut bacteria, it does not primarily absorb nutrients or produce digestive enzymes; those functions are mainly carried out by the small intestine. Thus, the statement is false.

20. Answer: B) Medulla oblongata

Explanation: The medulla oblongata, part of the brainstem, is responsible for regulating vital autonomic functions such as heart rate, blood pressure, and respiration. It is a crucial area for maintaining homeostasis. The cerebellum coordinates voluntary movements, the hypothalamus regulates body temperature, hunger, and other homeostatic processes, and the thalamus acts as a relay station for sensory information.

Medical Terminology in Phlebotomy

21. **Answer: C) Coagulation**

Explanation: Coagulation refers to the complex process where blood forms clots to prevent further bleeding after an injury. This involves platelets and clotting factors working together to form a stable clot. Hemostasis is a broader term that includes coagulation as a part of stopping blood flow, while hemolysis refers to the destruction of red blood cells, and erythropoiesis is the production of red blood cells.

22. Answer: B) Leukopenia

Explanation: Leukopenia describes a decrease in the number of white blood cells (leukocytes), which is critical for the body's immune defense against infections. A low white blood cell count can leave the patient vulnerable to infections, as there are fewer immune cells available to respond to pathogens. This condition can arise from various factors, including bone marrow disorders, autoimmune diseases, certain medications (such as chemotherapy), and viral infections. Understanding leukopenia is essential for monitoring the patient's immune status and developing strategies to minimize infection risk, such as prophylactic antibiotics or lifestyle modifications to reduce exposure to pathogens. In contrast, leukocytosis indicates an increase in white blood cells, often as a response to infection or stress, while thrombocytopenia pertains to low platelet counts, affecting clotting, and anemia refers to low red blood cell levels, impacting oxygen transport.

23. Answer: B) The percentage of red blood cells in the blood

Explanation: Hematocrit refers to the percentage of the volume of blood that is composed of red blood cells (RBCs). It is an important indicator of a person's red blood cell levels and can be used to diagnose and monitor conditions such as anemia, dehydration, and polycythemia. A low hematocrit value may indicate anemia, while a high value could suggest dehydration or polycythemia.

24. Answer: A) Phlebitis

Explanation: Phlebitis refers to the inflammation of a vein. It is often associated with pain, redness, and swelling in the affected area and can occur in superficial veins (superficial phlebitis) or deep veins (deep vein phlebitis, often linked to thrombosis). Phlebitis can be caused by injury, infection, or the presence of a blood clot.

Aseptic Techniques

25. Answer: C) 70% Isopropyl alcohol

Explanation: 70% isopropyl alcohol is the standard antiseptic used for routine venipuncture due to its effective antimicrobial properties. The 70% concentration allows for optimal penetration of the skin's surface, effectively killing bacteria and reducing the microbial load at the site. It evaporates quickly, minimizing irritation and allowing for a clean area for needle insertion. While iodine-based solutions and chlorhexidine gluconate are also effective, they are often reserved for situations requiring a higher level of antisepsis or in surgical settings. Hydrogen peroxide, while antiseptic, is not typically used for venipuncture because it can be harsh on tissues and may not effectively reduce bacteria in the same way as alcohol or chlorhexidine.

26. Answer: A) It ensures maximum effectiveness in killing microorganisms

Explanation: Allowing the antiseptic to dry ensures its maximum effectiveness in reducing microorganisms on the skin. Wet antiseptic can dilute the effectiveness and increase the risk of contamination. It also minimizes patient discomfort and reduces the chance of interference with the blood sample, though these are secondary benefits.

27. Answer: C) To destroy or inhibit microorganisms and prevent infection

Explanation: The primary purpose of using antiseptics during venipuncture is to destroy or inhibit microorganisms on the skin, thereby reducing the risk of introducing bacteria or other pathogens into the bloodstream. Proper skin antisepsis helps prevent infections at the puncture site or in the bloodstream, which is critical in medical procedures involving needle penetration.

28. Answer: C) Palpating the puncture site with bare hands after cleansing, which could introduce contaminants and negate the antiseptic effect

Explanation: Palpating the puncture site with bare hands after it has been cleansed is a breach of aseptic technique because it risks reintroducing bacteria and other pathogens that the cleaning process aimed to eliminate. The rationale behind this standard is to ensure that once a site has been sanitized, it remains free from external contamination until the procedure is completed.

29. Answer: B) Use both alcohol and povidone-iodine to cleanse the site

Explanation: When collecting blood cultures, the risk of contamination is higher, so a two-step process is required to clean the site. First, clean the area with 70% isopropyl alcohol, then apply povidone-iodine (or chlorhexidine) to reduce the skin's bacterial count further. This step minimizes the risk of introducing bacteria into the blood sample.

Explanation: The minimum recommended duration for handwashing to maintain aseptic conditions is at least 20 seconds. This duration is essential for effectively removing dirt, debris, and pathogens from the hands. Key factors that contribute to the effectiveness of handwashing include using soap and clean running water, ensuring all surfaces of the hands (including between fingers and under nails) are scrubbed, and rinsing thoroughly. Studies have shown that handwashing for less than 20 seconds may not adequately reduce the microbial load, increasing the risk of infection during invasive procedures such as venipuncture. Additionally, proper technique and the use of hand sanitizers when soap and water are not available further enhance hand hygiene practices in clinical settings.

31. Answer: B) Collecting blood from a patient with an active infectio

Explanation: Sterile gloves are critical in this scenario to prevent the introduction of additional pathogens into the bloodstream, particularly since the patient is already at risk of infection. Using non-sterile gloves could facilitate the transmission of harmful microorganisms, leading to complications such as systemic infection or sepsis.

32. Answer: B) To protect the healthcare worker from exposure to bloodborne pathogens

Explanation: The primary reason for wearing gloves during the entire phlebotomy procedure is to protect the healthcare worker from exposure to bloodborne pathogens, such as HIV, hepatitis B, and hepatitis C, that may be present in the patient's blood. Gloves act as a barrier between the healthcare worker and any potential contaminants.

33. Answer: B) By applying an antiseptic solution and allowing it to dry completely

Explanation: The phlebotomist should apply an antiseptic solution, such as 70% isopropyl alcohol or chlorhexidine gluconate, to the venipuncture site and allow it to dry completely. This practice is essential because it effectively reduces the microbial load on the skin, thereby minimizing the risk of infection during the procedure. Proper skin disinfection is a critical component of infection control in healthcare settings. Using a tourniquet alone does not address microbial contamination, while wiping the area with dry gauze does not provide adequate antiseptic action. Asking the patient to wash the site is not standard practice and may not achieve the necessary disinfection level. Ensuring effective skin preparation safeguards both the patient's health and the integrity of the procedure.

Phlebotomy and Vascular Anatomy

34. Answer: C) Median cubital vein, the preferred site for venipuncture because of its central location, size, and minimal risk of complications with surrounding structures

Explanation: The **median cubital vein** is the most commonly selected vein for venipuncture, primarily due to its optimal anatomical position in the antecubital fossa. Its central location allows for easier access, and it is generally larger in diameter compared to other veins in the area, facilitating successful blood draws. Additionally, its relatively superficial position minimizes the risk of damaging nearby nerves and arteries, making it the safest and most efficient choice for healthcare providers.

35. Answer: B) It is often more visible and easier to palpate in obese patients, facilitating access.

Explanation: The cephalic vein is frequently chosen for venipuncture in patients with higher BMI because it tends to be more visible and palpable, even when other veins are obscured by adipose tissue. This visibility makes it easier for the phlebotomist to locate and access the vein. While it is not the largest vein in the body (that distinction belongs to the vena cava), its larger size compared to other superficial veins and its outer location on the forearm enhance its accessibility. The cephalic vein's anatomical position is significant because it may also have branches that can complicate venipuncture if not properly assessed. Understanding these factors is crucial for effective and successful venipuncture, ensuring patient safety and quality of blood samples.

36. Answer: A) The basilic vein is located medial to the median cubital vein.

Explanation: In the antecubital fossa, the median cubital vein is typically situated centrally and is commonly used for venipuncture. The basilic vein runs along the medial side of the arm, making it medial to the median cubital vein. This anatomical relationship is important for healthcare providers when selecting veins for blood draws.

37. Answer: B) Higher likelihood of nerve damage

Explanation: The basilic vein is located near several important structures, including nerves. When puncturing the basilic vein, there is a higher risk of inadvertently damaging the median nerve, which runs in proximity to the vein. This could lead to complications such as pain, tingling, or loss of function in the affected area.

38. Answer: B) Great saphenous vein—Evaluate why this vein is preferred for venipuncture in the foot, considering its size, location, and the lower risk of complications compared to other veins.

Explanation: The **great saphenous vein** is most commonly selected for venipuncture on the foot due to its larger diameter and superficial location, making it easier to access while minimizing the risk of complications such as nerve damage or puncturing adjacent arteries. This vein runs along the medial aspect of the leg and is well-supported, which enhances its accessibility during the procedure.

39. Answer: B) It is located centrally and is typically more superficial than other veins.

Explanation: The median cubital vein is centrally located in the antecubital fossa and is often more superficial than the basilic and cephalic veins, making it easier to access. This position reduces the risk of complications and increases the likelihood of successful venipuncture. Its consistent location and size also contribute to its popularity as a venipuncture site.

40. Answer: A) Patient anatomy—Evaluate how variations in a patient's anatomy, such as obesity or previous venipuncture scars, might impact the visibility and accessibility of the median cubital vein compared to the cephalic vein.

Explanation: A phlebotomist may opt for the **cephalic vein** when anatomical variations make the **median cubital vein** difficult to palpate or visualize. In patients with obesity, for example, the deeper placement of the median cubital vein may hinder access, while the more superficial position of the cephalic vein can provide a viable alternative. Additionally, patients with a history of frequent venipuncture may have scarring that affects the median cubital vein, further necessitating the choice of the cephalic vein.

41. Answer: C) It may serve as a connection between the basilic and cephalic veins, providing alternative access points.

Explanation: The median antebrachial vein runs along the midline of the forearm and can serve as a connecting pathway between the basilic and cephalic veins. Its presence offers healthcare providers alternative access points for venipuncture, especially in cases where the median cubital vein is not accessible or suitable for blood draws.

42. Answer: C) The proximity of major nerves and arteries to the chosen vein—Discuss why understanding the anatomy of the area, particularly the location of major nerves and arteries, is vital for preventing complications.

Explanation: The **proximity of major nerves and arteries** to the chosen vein is the most critical anatomical consideration when selecting a venipuncture site. Knowledge of the vascular and nervous anatomy of the area helps phlebotomists avoid serious complications such as nerve damage, which can lead to chronic pain or dysfunction, and arterial puncture, which can result in excessive bleeding or hematoma formation.

Blood Components

43. Answer: A) Plasma contains clotting factors, while serum does not, making plasma suitable for coagulation studies.

Explanation: The key difference between plasma and serum is that plasma contains clotting factors, such as fibrinogen, while serum is the liquid portion of blood after clotting has occurred and is thus free of clotting factors. This distinction is critical when determining the type of diagnostic tests to perform. Plasma is typically used for coagulation studies, where the presence of clotting factors is necessary to measure how long it takes for blood to clot. Serum, on the other hand, is used in tests that do not require clotting factors, such as electrolyte panels, hormone levels, or certain antibody tests. Understanding this difference ensures proper sample handling and testing, which is essential for accurate diagnostic results in clinical settings.

44 .Answer: B) They help in the formation of blood clots to stop bleeding.

Explanation: The primary role of platelets is to contribute to **hemostasis**, which is the process of stopping bleeding. When a blood vessel is damaged, platelets quickly gather at the site, adhere to the vessel walls, and form a temporary "platelet plug." They also release chemical signals that attract other clotting factors, leading to the formation of a stable blood clot. This action prevents excessive blood loss and facilitates wound healing.

45. Answer: D) White blood cells

Explanation: White blood cells (leukocytes) are the primary cells involved in the body's immune response. They help fight infections by identifying and attacking pathogens such as bacteria, viruses, and other foreign invaders. There are several types of white blood cells, including neutrophils,

46. Answer: A) Plasma, buffy coat, red blood cells—Discuss the composition of each layer, including the importance of plasma for testing electrolytes, proteins, and hormones, the role of the buffy coat in evaluating immune function, and how red blood cells reflect oxygen-carrying capacity and anemia.

Explanation: When a blood sample is centrifuged, it typically separates into **plasma at the top**, the **buffy coat in the middle**, and **red blood cells at the bottom**. Plasma, which is the least dense component, contains water, electrolytes, proteins (like albumin and clotting factors), hormones, and waste products. It is essential for many clinical tests, including liver function tests and coagulation studies.

47. Answer: C) Bone marrow

Explanation: Red blood cells (RBCs) are produced in the bone marrow through a process called erythropoiesis. Once mature, they are released into the bloodstream to carry oxygen to tissues. Unlike some other cells, RBCs do not have a nucleus, allowing more space for hemoglobin, the protein responsible for oxygen transport. RBCs have a lifespan of about 120 days before being removed by the spleen.

48. Answer: B) False

Explanation: While the bicarbonate buffering system is crucial for maintaining blood pH balance, it does not operate in isolation. The system works in conjunction with the respiratory and renal systems. The respiratory system helps regulate pH by controlling carbon dioxide levels, which affects the concentration of carbonic acid in the blood. The renal system contributes by regulating the excretion and reabsorption of bicarbonate. Thus, the bicarbonate buffering system interacts with these other systems to maintain blood pH within the normal range.

49. Answer: A. The liquid portion of the blood that contains clotting factors

Explanation: Plasma is the liquid portion of the blood obtained when whole blood is treated with anticoagulants to prevent clotting. It contains clotting factors, electrolytes, hormones, and other proteins.

50. Answer: C) Clotting factors, which are required for coagulation tests

Explanation: Clotting factors, such as fibrinogen, are absent in serum because they are consumed during the clotting process when blood is allowed to clot. This makes serum distinct from plasma, which retains clotting factors when anticoagulants are used. The absence of clotting factors in serum is crucial for tests where these proteins could interfere, such as certain metabolic or immunological assays. Plasma, however, is used for tests like coagulation studies, where the presence of clotting factors is necessary to assess blood clotting function. Understanding the differences in the composition of serum and plasma helps guide the selection of the appropriate specimen for accurate diagnostic results.

51. Answer: C) Polycythemia

Explanation: Polycythemia is a condition characterized by an elevated number of red blood cells (erythrocytes) in the blood. This can increase the blood's viscosity, making it thicker and potentially leading to complications like blood clots, hypertension, and increased risk of stroke. Polycythemia can be primary (due to bone marrow overproduction) or secondary (due to factors like low oxygen levels).

52. Answer: C) To engulf and destroy bacteria and other pathogens

Explanation: The primary function of **neutrophils** is to act as the body's first line of defense against bacterial infections. They are a type of phagocyte, meaning they engulf (phagocytose) and destroy invading pathogens like bacteria and fungi. When an infection occurs, neutrophils are among the first immune cells to arrive at the site of infection, where they ingest and neutralize harmful microorganisms.

53. Answer: C) To form a mesh that stabilizes the platelet plug—Discuss the transformation of fibrinogen into fibrin, how it creates a mesh-like network, and its importance in reinforcing the platelet plug to prevent blood loss.

Explanation: Fibrin plays a vital role in the **final stages of hemostasis** by forming a **mesh** that stabilizes the platelet plug at the site of injury. This occurs when the enzyme thrombin converts **fibrinogen**, a soluble protein in the blood, into **fibrin**, an insoluble protein. The fibrin strands interlace with the platelets, creating a stable and durable clot that seals the damaged vessel, preventing further bleeding.

54. Answer: A) True

Explanation: The PT test evaluates the extrinsic and common coagulation pathways, not the intrinsic pathway. An elevated PT can indeed indicate various issues including liver disease, vitamin K deficiency, and the impact of anticoagulant medications. This makes the PT test an important tool for assessing overall coagulation function and managing therapeutic interventions.

55. Answer: C) It filters and removes old or damaged red blood cells, recycling iron and preventing accumulation of dysfunctional cells.

Explanation: The spleen's primary role in red blood cell management is filtering out old, damaged, or abnormal red blood cells from the bloodstream. This process is essential for maintaining healthy circulation, as it ensures that only functional red blood cells, which can effectively transport oxygen, remain in circulation. The spleen also recycles valuable components, such as iron, from the degraded red blood cells for reuse in new red blood cell production. In adults, red blood cell production occurs primarily in the bone marrow, and while the spleen can store small amounts of blood, its storage capacity is not the primary function. Understanding this process is crucial in diagnosing and managing conditions like hemolytic anemia, where the spleen may become overactive in destroying red blood cells, or in cases of splenomegaly, where the spleen's size increases due to excess filtration activity.

56. Answer: B) It increases the risk of abnormal blood clot formation.

Explanation: Thrombocytosis is a condition characterized by an abnormally high number of platelets in the blood. While platelets are essential for normal blood clotting, an elevated count can increase the risk of forming abnormal blood clots (thrombosis) within blood vessels. This can lead to complications such as deep vein thrombosis (DVT), pulmonary embolism, stroke, or heart attack, depending on where the clot forms.

57. Answer: B) Eosinophils

Explanation: Eosinophils are a type of white blood cell that play a key role in the body's immune response, particularly during allergic reactions and asthma. These cells are involved in the inflammatory processes by releasing substances like histamines that contribute to the symptoms of allergic conditions. Elevated eosinophil levels are commonly seen in conditions like asthma, hay fever, and other allergic disorders.

Blood Group Systems

58. Answer: A) ABO system

Explanation: The ABO blood group system is determined by the presence or absence of A and B antigens on the surface of red blood cells. The four main blood types in this system are A (with A antigen), B (with B antigen), AB (with both A and B antigens), and O (with neither antigen). The ABO system is crucial in blood transfusion compatibility, as receiving blood with incompatible antigens can trigger an immune response.

59. Answer: B) It affects whether a blood transfusion will result in an immune reaction.

Explanation: The **Rh factor** (Rhesus factor) is an antigen present on the surface of red blood cells. The presence or absence of the Rh factor determines whether someone is **Rh-positive** (Rh+) or **Rh-negative** (Rh−). In blood transfusion, if Rh-positive blood is given to an Rh-negative individual, the recipient's immune system may recognize the Rh antigen as foreign and produce antibodies, leading to an immune reaction, which can be serious or even life-threatening.

60. Answer: D) All blood types—Explain why AB positive patients are considered universal recipients, focusing on the absence of anti-A, anti-B, and anti-Rh antibodies, and the immunological compatibility with all blood types.

Explanation: Patients with **AB positive blood** can receive blood from all types—**O, A, B, and AB**, both positive and negative—due to the absence of antibodies against the A and B antigens.

Additionally, being **Rh-positive** allows them to receive both **Rh-positive** and **Rh-negative** blood. The immunological mechanism behind this compatibility is that their immune system does not react to any ABO or Rh antigens present in the donor blood, making transfusion reactions highly unlikely.

61. Answer: B) Type O negative blood

Explanation: Individuals with type O negative blood are considered universal donors but can only receive type O negative blood. This is because O negative blood lacks A, B, and Rh antigens, meaning any transfusion containing these antigens (such as A, B, or Rh-positive blood) could trigger an immune response.

62. Answer: A) True

Explanation: The Rh system is indeed a critical component of blood typing. The Rh factor (Rhesus factor) is a specific antigen present on the surface of red blood cells. Individuals who have this antigen are classified as Rh-positive, while those who lack the antigen are classified as Rh-negative. This classification is important for compatibility in blood transfusions and pregnancy, as Rh incompatibility between mother and fetus can lead to complications.

63. Answer: C) HLA

Explanation: The **HLA system** (Human Leukocyte Antigen) is primarily involved in organ and tissue transplantation, as it helps the immune system differentiate between self and non-self cells. It is **not commonly used in blood transfusions**. Instead, it plays a major role in matching donors and recipients in organ transplants to prevent rejection.

64. Answer: B) Ensuring the patient and donor blood types are compatible—Analyze how the compatibility of ABO and Rh antigens plays a pivotal role in avoiding dangerous transfusion reactions, and discuss the implications of undetected incompatibilities.

Explanation: The most critical aspect of a **crossmatch test** is confirming **blood type compatibility**, specifically between the **ABO** and **Rh systems**. Crossmatching ensures that the recipient's immune system will not attack the donor's red blood cells, which could lead to a **hemolytic transfusion reaction**. Such a reaction can be life-threatening, as the immune system destroys incompatible red blood cells, leading to complications like shock, kidney failure, and even death.

65. Answer: B) Hemolytic transfusion reaction

Explanation: A patient with **type B positive blood** has B antigens on their red blood cells and anti-A antibodies in their plasma. If this patient receives **type A positive blood**, the **anti-A antibodies** in their blood will recognize the A antigens on the donor red blood cells as foreign and mount an immune response. This can lead to a **hemolytic transfusion reaction**, where the patient's immune system attacks and destroys the transfused red blood cells. Hemolytic reactions can cause serious complications such as fever, chills, kidney failure, or even death.

66. Answer: B) It can lead to hemolytic transfusion reactions if incompatible blood is transfused.

Explanation: The **Kell blood group system** consists of several antigens (e.g., K and k) present on the surface of red blood cells. If a patient who has anti-K antibodies receives blood that has the K antigen (K+), it can result in a hemolytic transfusion reaction, where the recipient's immune system attacks the transfused red blood cells. This reaction can lead to serious complications, including fever, chills, and kidney damage.

67. Answer: B) Rh incompatibility—Discuss the mechanism of Rh incompatibility, focusing on how the Rh-negative mother's immune system may produce antibodies against the Rh-positive baby's red blood cells, leading to hemolytic disease of the

newborn (HDN), and the role of RhoGAM in preventing this condition.

Explanation: The most significant concern is **Rh incompatibility**, where the Rh-negative mother's immune system may become sensitized to Rh-positive blood cells from the baby. This can happen during pregnancy or delivery if fetal blood cells enter the mother's bloodstream, prompting the mother's immune system to produce antibodies that target the baby's Rh-positive red blood cells. This immune response can cause **hemolytic disease of the newborn (HDN)**, leading to anemia, jaundice, or severe complications in the baby.

68. Answer: C) Rh factor

Explanation: A patient with type B negative blood does not have the Rh antigen. If they receive type B positive blood, which contains the Rh factor, their immune system may recognize the Rh antigen as foreign and develop antibodies against it. This could result in an immune response, leading to complications such as a hemolytic transfusion reaction.

69. Answer: A) The patient is at risk of developing hemolytic disease of the fetus and newborn (HDFN) if the fetus expresses the K antigen, requiring close monitoring.

Explanation: The Kell blood group system includes antigens like K (Kell) and k (cellano), which are significant in both transfusion reactions and pregnancies. If a pregnant woman develops anti-K antibodies and the fetus inherits the K antigen from the father, these antibodies can cross the placenta and attack the fetal red blood cells, leading to **hemolytic disease of the fetus and newborn (HDFN).** This can cause anemia, jaundice, or more severe complications like hydrops fetalis. To manage this, clinicians may perform regular monitoring through Doppler ultrasound to assess fetal anemia and, in severe cases, intrauterine transfusions may be necessary. Unlike Rh antibodies, the Kell system is less frequently discussed but equally important in transfusion and prenatal care decisions.

70. Answer: B) Type A individuals have anti-B antibodies present in their plasma.

Explanation: In the ABO blood group system, individuals naturally produce antibodies against the antigens they lack. For example, individuals with **type A blood** have A antigens on their red blood cells and will produce **anti-B antibodies** in their plasma, which target B antigens.

71. Answer: B) Anti-A serum—Discuss how this reagent interacts with A antigens on the red blood cell surface and the significance of agglutination in confirming blood type.

Explanation: The reagent **Anti-A serum** is specifically designed to detect the presence of **A antigens** on the surface of red blood cells. When a sample of blood is mixed with Anti-A serum, the serum contains antibodies that bind to any A antigens present. If agglutination occurs (clumping of red blood cells), it indicates that the blood type is either A or AB, as those blood types express A antigens.

72. Answer: C) To assess the compatibility between the donor's red blood cells and the recipient's plasma.

Explanation: The primary goal of a **crossmatch test** is to ensure that the **donor's red blood cells** are compatible with the **recipient's plasma**. This test helps identify any potential immune reactions that may occur due to incompatibility, particularly with respect to ABO and Rh blood group antigens. A successful crossmatch indicates that the blood transfusion is likely to proceed without adverse reactions.

73. Answer: B) Rho(D) immune globulin (RhIg)

Explanation: Rho(D) immune globulin (RhIg) is administered to Rh-negative pregnant women who are carrying an Rh-positive baby. This treatment works by preventing the mother's immune system from producing antibodies against the Rh-positive blood cells of the fetus. If the mother is sensitized (has already formed anti-Rh antibodies), RhIg will not be effective, but administering it during and after pregnancy can prevent sensitization in future pregnancies.

Capillary Puncture

74. Answer: C) Proper warming of the site prior to puncture

Explanation: Proper warming of the site prior to puncture is crucial because it increases blood flow to the area, leading to a larger and more adequate blood sample. Warming helps ensure that the capillary beds are filled, reducing the likelihood of obtaining interstitial fluid, which can dilute the blood sample and lead to inaccurate test results.

75. Answer: B) 2-3 mm

Explanation: The appropriate depth for a capillary puncture on an infant is typically **2-3 mm**. This depth is sufficient to penetrate the skin and reach the capillary beds without risking injury to underlying structures, such as nerves or bones.

76. Answer: C) The risk of damaging the nerves in the finger is higher in infants, making the heelstick a safer option that reduces the risk of long-term nerve injury.

Explanation: The primary reason for selecting a heelstick over a fingerstick in infants is the lower risk of nerve damage. Infants' fingers are much smaller and contain a higher concentration of nerves relative to their size, meaning a fingerstick could result in nerve injury, which could impair function or sensation in the hand. The heel, particularly in the areas typically used for heelsticks, has fewer critical nerves, reducing the risk of causing nerve damage. This ensures that blood collection is safe and minimizes the chances of long-term complications. While other factors, such as the presence of capillaries and discomfort, may also play a role, preventing nerve injury is the most significant concern.

77. Answer: A) Hematoma formation

Explanation: Hematoma formation is a common complication that can occur during or after a capillary puncture, particularly if the puncture site is not properly managed or if excessive pressure is applied after the puncture. A hematoma forms when blood leaks from the capillaries into the surrounding tissue, leading to swelling and discoloration.

78. Answer: B) Middle finger—Analyze why the middle finger is typically preferred for capillary puncture, considering anatomical factors such as blood flow, size, and patient comfort.

Explanation: The **middle finger** is preferred for capillary puncture in older children and adults because it offers a combination of good blood flow and a larger surface area, which facilitates easier access and a more efficient sample collection. The middle finger generally has fewer sensory nerve endings compared to the thumb and index finger, reducing discomfort during the puncture.

79. Answer: B) False

Explanation: It is not recommended to puncture the same site multiple times during a capillary puncture procedure. Doing so can cause discomfort, tissue damage, and potentially affect the accuracy of the test results. If the initial puncture is unsuccessful or if there are complications, it is better to select a new site for the puncture rather than re-puncturing the same area.

80. Answer: B) Fragile veins or is a young child

Explanation: Capillary puncture is used when venipuncture may be difficult, such as in patients with fragile veins (common in the elderly) or young children. It is also used when only a small amount of blood is needed, such as for glucose or hemoglobin testing. Venipuncture is generally preferred when largr volumes of blood are required or when specific tests, such as blood cultures, are needed.

81. Answer: A) Presence of a rash or skin infection

Explanation: A **rash or skin infection** at the puncture site makes it unsuitable for a capillary puncture because it increases the risk of infection and may compromise the quality of the blood sample. Using an infected site could introduce pathogens into the bloodstream.

82. Answer: C) Capillary blood, which is a mixture of arterial and venous blood and can be used for rapid testing but may yield different results compared to venous blood.

Explanation: Capillary puncture typically yields **capillary blood**, which is a mixture of arterial and venous blood, as well as interstitial fluid. This method is favored for its convenience and speed, especially for point-of-care testing, such as blood glucose monitoring or infant screening tests. However, the composition of capillary blood can affect the accuracy of certain laboratory tests; for instance, capillary blood may have different levels of certain analytes compared to venous blood due to the mixing of blood types and the influence of tissue fluid. Understanding these differences is crucial for interpreting test results accurately, particularly in clinical scenarios where precise measurements are essential.

83. Answer: B) To collect blood samples for laboratory analysis—Discuss the advantages of using capillary tubes for sample collection, including their appropriateness for specific tests and situations, and how they facilitate the collection of small blood volumes.

Explanation: Capillary tubes are primarily used for collecting small volumes of blood during a **capillary puncture**, making them ideal for tests where only a few drops of blood are needed. This method is particularly beneficial for infants, young children, or patients with difficult venous access.

84. Answer: B) 30-45 degrees

Explanation: The recommended angle for making a capillary puncture is **30-45 degrees**. This angle allows for a clean puncture that effectively accesses the capillary bed while minimizing the risk of damage to underlying tissues and ensuring an adequate blood flow.

85. Answer: B) In a sharps container

Explanation: A used lancet should be disposed of in a **sharps container**. Sharps containers are specifically designed to safely contain used needles and other sharp instruments to prevent injury and reduce the risk of infection.

86. Answer: A) Excessive squeezing

Explanation: Applying excessive pressure or squeezing to the puncture site during a capillary blood collection can lead to the dilution of the sample with interstitial fluid, potentially compromising the test result's accuracy. It's important to use gentle pressure to collect a clean sample. Other factors, such as improper cleaning or patient identification, are important but do not directly affect the sample integrity in the same way.

87. Answer: C) To assess the percentage of red blood cells in the blood sample

Explanation: The primary purpose of the **microhematocrit tube** is to assess the **percentage of red blood cells (RBCs)** in a given volume of blood, commonly referred to as the hematocrit value. This measurement is crucial for evaluating conditions such as anemia, dehydration, and polycythemia.

88. Answer: B) Use an antiseptic wipe and allow it to dry completely

Explanation: Using an **antiseptic wipe** to clean the puncture site is the best method to ensure it is free of contamination. Allowing the antiseptic to dry completely is crucial because it helps kill any potential pathogens on the skin and reduces the risk of contamination during the puncture.

89. Answer: C) Vena cava

Explanation: The superior and inferior vena cavae are large veins that return deoxygenated blood from the body to the right atrium of the heart. The superior vena cava drains blood from the upper body, while the inferior vena cava drains blood from the lower body.

90. Answer: B) To generate electrical impulses that initiate the heart's contraction

Explanation: The sinoatrial (SA) node, located in the right atrium, is often referred to as the heart's natural pacemaker. It generates electrical impulses that cause the atria to contract, sending blood into the ventricles. These impulses then travel to the atrioventricular (AV) node and throughout the heart, coordinating the heartbeat.

91. Answer: B) The thick muscular walls of arteries allow for regulation of blood flow and pressure.

Explanation: The patient's symptoms of intermittent claudication suggest peripheral artery disease (PAD), which is often caused by atherosclerosis leading to narrowed arteries. Arteries have thick, muscular walls that enable them to withstand and regulate the high pressure of blood pumped from the heart. This characteristic allows for vasodilation and vasoconstriction, which is critical in managing blood flow to various tissues, especially in the context of conditions like PAD.

92. Answer: A) Right atrium → Right ventricle → Pulmonary artery → Lungs → Left atrium → Left ventricle → Aorta

Explanation: This sequence accurately describes the pathway of deoxygenated blood returning to the heart, being pumped to the lungs for oxygenation, and then returning as oxygenated blood to be distributed throughout the body.

93. Answer: B) "Lub" is produced by the closure of the atrioventricular (AV) valves, and "dub" is produced by the closure of the semilunar valves.

Explanation: The "lub" sound (S1) occurs when the atrioventricular valves (the mitral and tricuspid valves) close at the beginning of ventricular contraction (systole). The "dub" sound (S2) occurs when the semilunar valves (the aortic and pulmonary valves) close at the end of ventricular contraction, marking the beginning of diastole.

94. Answer: B) "Lub" is produced by the closure of the atrioventricular (AV) valves, and "dub" is produced by the closure of the semilunar valves.

Explanation: The "lub" sound (S1) occurs when the atrioventricular valves (the mitral and tricuspid valves) close at the beginning of ventricular contraction (systole). The "dub" sound (S2) occurs when the semilunar valves (the aortic and pulmonary valves) close at the end of ventricular contraction, marking the beginning of diastole.

95. Answer: B) QRS complex

Explanation: The QRS complex on an EKG tracing represents the depolarization of the ventricles. This phase is critical as it indicates the electrical activation of the ventricles, leading to ventricular contraction and the pumping of blood to the lungs and the rest of the body.

96. Answer: C) To return deoxygenated blood from the upper body to the right atrium of the heart.

Explanation: The superior vena cava is a large vein that collects deoxygenated blood from the upper half of the body (including the head, neck, arms, and upper trunk) and returns it to the right atrium of the heart. This function is crucial in the circulatory system, as it ensures that deoxygenated blood is directed to the heart for reoxygenation in the lungs.

97. Answer: B) The AV node serves as a delay point for electrical impulses, allowing for

coordinated contraction of the atria and ventricles.

Explanation: The atrioventricular (AV) node is crucial in the heart's electrical conduction system. It receives electrical impulses from the atria and introduces a delay before transmitting them to the ventricles. This delay ensures that the atria contract and empty blood into the ventricles before the ventricles contract, promoting efficient pumping of blood.

98. Answer: B) To prevent the atrioventricular valves from inverting during ventricular contraction.

Explanation: The chordae tendineae are fibrous cords that connect the papillary muscles to the atrioventricular (AV) valves (mitral and tricuspid valves). Their primary role is to prevent the valves from prolapsing or inverting into the atria when the ventricles contract (systole). This ensures that blood flows in the correct direction—from the atria to the ventricles and not back into the atria.

99. Answer: C) **Ventricular repolarization, indicating the recovery phase of the ventricles after contraction.**

Explanation: The T wave on an EKG tracing represents the repolarization of the ventricles. This phase occurs after the ventricles have contracted and is critical for restoring the resting state of the myocardial cells, preparing them for the next contraction. Abnormalities in the T wave can indicate issues such as electrolyte imbalances, ischemia, or other cardiac conditions.

100. Answer: C) **The heart muscle relaxes, and the chambers fill with blood from the atria.**

Explanation: Diastole is the phase of the cardiac cycle during which the heart muscle relaxes, allowing the atria and ventricles to fill with blood. During this time, the atrioventricular valves (mitral and tricuspid) are open, facilitating the flow of blood from the atria into the ventricles.

101. Answer: A) During atrial fibrillation, the left atrium experiences ineffective contractions, leading to stasis of blood and an increased risk of thrombus formation.

Explanation: In atrial fibrillation, the normal rhythmic contraction of the left atrium is disrupted, leading to ineffective blood flow and stasis. This stasis significantly increases the risk of thrombus (blood clot) formation, which can result in serious complications such as stroke.

102. Answer: B) During ventricular systole, the ventricles contract vigorously, resulting in increased intraventricular pressure that closes the AV valves and ejects blood into the systemic and pulmonary circulation, which is vital for delivering oxygen and nutrients to tissues.

Explanation: Ventricular systole is crucial as it involves the forceful contraction of the ventricles, generating pressure that ensures the effective ejection of blood into both the aorta and pulmonary artery. This process is essential for maintaining adequate perfusion of oxygenated blood to the body's tissues and organs, underscoring its importance in overall cardiovascular health.

103. Answer: B) Dysfunctional capillaries may hinder the diffusion of oxygen from the blood into the tissues, resulting in decreased oxygen availability and subsequent fatigue.

Explanation: In the context of the cardiovascular system, capillaries are crucial for efficient gas exchange and nutrient delivery. If capillary function is impaired—due to conditions such as inflammation, endothelial dysfunction, or structural abnormalities—oxygen may not diffuse effectively from the blood into the tissues. This results in hypoxia (insufficient oxygen levels in tissues), leading to symptoms such as fatigue, weakness, and decreased exercise tolerance.

Hemostasis and the Coagulation

104. Answer: C) Factor IX; its deficiency can cause hemophilia B, resulting in severe bleeding episodes despite normal levels of other factors.

Explanation: In the context of the intrinsic pathway of coagulation, Factor IX is essential for effective clot formation. Its deficiency leads to hemophilia B, a genetic bleeding disorder characterized by prolonged bleeding episodes, especially after injury or surgery.

105. Answer: C) Vitamin K

Explanation: Vitamin K is crucial for the synthesis of several key clotting factors (II, VII, IX, and X) in the liver, enabling the proper functioning of the coagulation cascade. A deficiency in vitamin K can significantly impair the synthesis of these clotting factors, resulting in an increased risk of bleeding disorders, such as easy bruising, prolonged bleeding from guts, and potentially severe hemorrhage in more serious cases. Monitoring vitamin K levels and ensuring adequate dietary intake (found in leafy greens and certain oils) is essential in managing patients with coagulation disorders or those on anticoagulant therapy, as vitamin K can influence the effectiveness of these medications.

106. Answer: B) Elevated D-dimer levels suggest active clot formation and breakdown, prompting further investigation for conditions like deep vein thrombosis (DVT) or pulmonary embolism (PE).

Explanation: Elevated D-dimer levels indicate the presence of fibrin degradation products in the blood, which occur during the breakdown of clots formed through the coagulation process. This elevation suggests that there may be ongoing thrombotic activity, which is critical in evaluating patients for conditions such as DVT or PE. While elevated D-dimer results do not provide a definitive diagnosis, they serve as a sensitive marker that prompts further diagnostic testing, such as imaging studies (e.g., ultrasound or CT scan), to confirm or rule out the presence of thrombosis. Understanding the implications of D-dimer levels in relation to coagulation is essential for appropriate clinical management and patient care.

107. Answer: C) Warfarin inhibits vitamin K-dependent clotting factors, reducing the synthesis of factors II, VII, IX, and X, which requires regular monitoring of INR for dosage adjustments.

Explanation: Warfarin acts by inhibiting the synthesis of vitamin K-dependent clotting factors in the liver, which include factors II (prothrombin), VII, IX, and X. This inhibition decreases the blood's ability to clot, making warfarin effective in preventing thromboembolic events in patients with conditions like atrial fibrillation. Due to its narrow therapeutic range and variability in patient response, regular monitoring of the INR is essential to ensure that the patient remains within the therapeutic range, balancing the risk of thrombosis against the risk of bleeding. Additionally, patients on warfarin need to be educated about dietary vitamin K intake, potential drug interactions, and signs of bleeding.

108. Answer: B) Forming a platelet plug

Explanation: Platelets play a vital role in hemostasis by quickly responding to blood vessel injury. They adhere to the damaged area and aggregate to form a temporary platelet plug, while also releasing chemicals that activate the coagulation cascade, ultimately leading to stable clot formation. Unlike red blood cells, platelets do not carry oxygen, nor do they produce antibodies or break down clots.

109. Answer: A) True

Explanation: The platelet aggregation test evaluates the ability of platelets to aggregate or clump together in response to specific substances called agonists. This test is crucial for diagnosing platelet disorders and assessing the functionality of platelets in the clotting process. Other tests that may be used include the platelet function analyzer (PFA-100) and the bleeding time test, but platelet aggregation remains a primary method for assessing platelet function.

110. Answer: B) Secondary hemostasis—Analyze how the conversion of prothrombin to thrombin signifies a shift from primary to secondary hemostasis, detailing the cascade of reactions that lead to clot stabilization and the role of thrombin in activating additional clotting factors.

Explanation: The conversion of **prothrombin to thrombin** occurs during **secondary hemostasis**. This phase is crucial for the stabilization of the initial platelet plug formed during primary hemostasis. Thrombin, once activated, not only converts fibrinogen into fibrin, forming a mesh that strengthens the platelet plug, but it also activates several other coagulation factors, amplifying the clotting response.

111. Answer: C) Thrombin converts fibrinogen to fibrin and activates platelets, thereby amplifying

the coagulation cascade and promoting stable clot formation.

Explanation: Thrombin is a crucial enzyme in the coagulation process with multiple functions. Its primary role is to convert fibrinogen, a soluble plasma protein, into insoluble fibrin strands, which form the backbone of a blood clot. Additionally, thrombin activates platelets, promoting their aggregation and further enhancing the coagulation cascade. This amplification effect is vital for effective hemostasis, ensuring that a stable and robust clot forms at the site of injury. Understanding the multifaceted role of thrombin is essential for clinicians managing patients with bleeding disorders or those requiring anticoagulation therapy.

112. Answer: B) Hemophilia

Explanation: Hemophilia is a genetic disorder where the body lacks certain clotting factors, leading to a higher risk of uncontrolled bleeding from minor injuries. While conditions like thrombocytopenia involve low platelet counts and can also result in bleeding issues, hemophilia specifically refers to the absence or deficiency of clotting factors essential for proper blood coagulation. Leukemia and polycythemia vera affect blood cell production but are not primarily linked to clotting factor deficiencies.

113. Answer: C) They facilitate the conversion of prothrombin to thrombin

Explanation: Calcium ions (Ca^{2+}) are essential cofactors in the coagulation cascade, particularly in facilitating the conversion of **prothrombin to thrombin**. This conversion is a pivotal step in secondary hemostasis. Calcium ions help bridge the interactions between clotting factors and activate several factors in the intrinsic and extrinsic pathways of coagulation.

114.Answer: B) Prolongation of aPTT primarily indicates a deficiency in the intrinsic pathway or the common pathway, possibly due to deficiencies

in Factors VIII, IX, XI, or XII, which may lead to hemophilia-like symptoms.

Explanation: The activated partial thromboplastin time (aPTT) specifically assesses the intrinsic and common pathways of the coagulation cascade. A prolonged aPTT indicates potential deficiencies in the factors associated with these pathways.

115. Answer: B) Endothelial injury exposes collagen, which activates Factor XII, leading to a cascade of reactions involving factors XI, IX, and VIII, ultimately forming a fibrin clot.

Explanation: The intrinsic pathway is initiated by endothelial injury, where exposure of collagen activates Factor XII upon contact. This starts a cascade that involves Factor XI, which then activates Factor IX. Factor IX, in conjunction with Factor VIII, activates Factor X, leading to the formation of thrombin and ultimately the conversion of fibrinogen to fibrin, resulting in clot formation.

116. Answer: B) Thrombophilia

Explanation: Thrombophilia is a condition that predisposes individuals to an increased risk of forming abnormal blood clots in veins or arteries. It can be inherited (such as Factor V Leiden mutation or prothrombin gene mutation) or acquired (due to conditions like antiphospholipid syndrome, certain cancers, or prolonged immobility). In this scenario, the patient's history of recurrent DVT and family predisposition suggests a hypercoagulable state, which is characteristic of thrombophilia. Recognizing this condition is critical for appropriate management, including anticoagulation therapy and lifestyle modifications to reduce the risk of future thrombotic events.

117. Answer: A) Sodium citrate

Explanation: Sodium citrate is the anticoagulant of choice for coagulation testing because it effectively binds free calcium ions in the blood. Calcium is a crucial cofactor in several steps of the coagulation cascade, so its removal prevents clot formation, enabling accurate assessment of clotting times like PT and aPTT. This is essential for diagnosing bleeding disorders, monitoring anticoagulant therapy, and conducting other coagulation studies. Understanding the specific function and application of sodium citrate is vital for laboratory professionals involved in hematology and coagulation diagnostics.

118. Answer: D) Hemoglobin

Explanation: Hemoglobin is the protein responsible for carrying oxygen in red blood cells and is not part of the coagulation cascade. In contrast, proteins such as Factor VII, fibrinogen, and thrombin are crucial components of the cascade, contributing to blood clot formation and the hemostatic process.

Laboratory Operations

119. Answer: B) The centrifuge separates the blood components based on their density, allowing for the isolation of plasma and cellular elements necessary for various tests.

Explanation: In the context of blood analysis, the **primary function of the centrifuge** is to separate the blood components—specifically, to isolate plasma from red blood cells and other cellular elements. By spinning the blood sample at high speeds, the centrifuge creates a centrifugal force that causes denser components (like red blood cells) to settle at the bottom of the tube, while the less dense plasma remains on top. This separation is crucial for many laboratory tests, such as biochemical assays, blood typing, and hematology analyses, as it allows for the specific examination of each component. Understanding the centrifuge's role in sample preparation is essential for laboratory technicians to ensure accurate and reliable test results.

120. Answer: B) Monitor long-term blood glucose control

Explanation: The HbA1c test measures the percentage of glycated hemoglobin, reflecting average blood glucose levels over the previous two to three months. It is a key tool in managing diabetes, helping healthcare providers evaluate how well blood sugar is being controlled. This test is not used for diagnosing anemia, assessing liver function, or measuring blood oxygen levels.

121. Answer: B) Insert the needle at a 15-30 degree angle and draw blood quickly

Explanation: The needle should be inserted at a 15-30 degree angle to ensure it enters the vein properly and minimizes discomfort for the patient. Drawing blood quickly helps in avoiding hemolysis and ensures an adequate sample. A 45-degree angle is too steep, and inserting the needle parallel or perpendicular to the vein can increase the risk of missing the vein or causing unnecessary trauma.

122. Answer: B) Filling tubes to the specified level

Explanation: Properly filling tubes to the specified level ensures the correct ratio of blood to anticoagulant or preservative, which is critical for accurate test results. Using the same needle for multiple draws can lead to contamination, shaking tubes vigorously can cause hemolysis, and allowing samples to sit at room temperature for too long can lead to degradation of the sample.

123. Answer: B) Urine

Explanation: Culture and sensitivity tests are commonly performed on urine samples to identify bacterial infections and determine the most effective antibiotics for treatment. Serum, plasma, and whole blood are used for other types of tests and analyses, but not typically for culture and sensitivity.

124. Answer: A) True

Explanation: Sodium citrate is indeed the standard additive used in blood collection tubes for coagulation tests. It functions as an anticoagulant by binding calcium ions, which are crucial for the clotting cascade. By removing calcium, sodium citrate prevents the blood from clotting inside the tube, allowing for accurate assessment of coagulation factors and tests such as PT (prothrombin time) and aPTT (activated partial thromboplastin time).

125. Answer: B) False

Explanation: According to CLSI guidelines, the correct order of draw starts with blood culture bottles (or sterile bottles), followed by the light blue top tube, then the red top tube, gold or tiger top tube, green top tube, purple or lavender top tube, and finally the gray top tube. The sequence is designed to prevent cross-contamination of additives and ensure the accuracy of test results. The light blue top tube should be drawn before the red top tube, not after.

126. Answer: B) Basic metabolic panel (BMP)

Explanation: The **Basic Metabolic Panel (BMP)** is primarily performed using a serum sample due to the need for accurate measurements of various analytes, including electrolytes, glucose, and kidney function indicators. Serum, obtained after blood has clotted and the cells have been removed, provides a clear liquid that is free from cellular components, allowing for precise analysis. This is particularly important for assessing metabolic processes and electrolyte balance, which can significantly influence patient care decisions. In contrast, tests like the CBC require whole blood to measure blood cell counts and types, while coagulation studies utilize plasma to evaluate the clotting ability of blood. Understanding the rationale behind the choice of sample type is crucial for laboratory professionals to ensure accurate and reliable diagnostic outcomes.

127. Answer: B) Thrombocytopenia

Explanation: Thrombocytopenia indicates a lower than normal platelet count in the blood, which can impair the body's ability to form clots and stop bleeding. In contrast, thrombocytosis refers to an elevated platelet count, hemophilia is related to deficiencies in clotting factors, and leukopenia refers to a low white blood cell count.

128. Answer: B) A localized collection of blood outside of blood vessels, typically due to injury or trauma.

Explanation: A hematoma is defined as a localized collection of blood that forms outside of blood vessels, usually as a result of trauma, injury, or bleeding disorders. It occurs when blood leaks from damaged vessels into surrounding tissues, leading to swelling and discoloration. Hematomas can vary in size and severity, and while small hematomas may resolve on their own, larger ones may require medical attention to prevent complications. Understanding hematomas is essential for healthcare professionals in assessing injuries and managing patient care.

129. Answer: B) Polycythemia occurs when there is an abnormal increase in red blood cells, which can thicken the blood and increase the risk of complications like clots, strokes, or heart attacks.

Explanation: Polycythemia is a condition marked by an excessive number of red blood cells (RBCs) in circulation, which leads to the thickening of the blood. This increased viscosity can raise the risk of cardiovascular complications, such as blood clots, strokes, and heart attacks. The condition can occur due to genetic mutations affecting the bone marrow (primary polycythemia) or as a response to low oxygen levels (secondary polycythemia). Understanding the underlying causes and potential risks associated with polycythemia is critical for medical professionals when diagnosing and managing this disorder.

130. Answer: B) Arteriosclerosis results in the thickening and hardening of the arterial walls due to calcium deposition, reduced elasticity, and narrowed vessel lumen, increasing the risk of ischemia and tissue necrosis.

Explanation: Arteriosclerosis refers to the hardening and thickening of the arterial walls, often due to calcium deposition and the loss of arterial elasticity. This reduces the vessel's ability to dilate properly, leading to decreased blood flow to tissues. As a result, patients may experience **intermittent claudication** (leg pain during walking) due to insufficient blood supply, and untreated arteriosclerosis can progress to more severe conditions like tissue ischemia, gangrene, heart attacks, and strokes.

131. Answer: C) Increase in cell count—Discuss how "-cytosis" indicates an increase in the number of specific cell types, including possible causes such as infection, inflammation, or malignancy, and explain how this affects diagnostic and therapeutic decisions.

Explanation: The suffix **"-cytosis"** indicates an **increase in the number of cells** and is often seen in conditions where certain blood cells proliferate beyond normal levels. For example, **leukocytosis** refers to an elevated white blood cell count, which can be a sign of infection, inflammation, or in some cases, leukemia. Similarly, **erythrocytosis** refers to an abnormally high red blood cell count, which can result from polycythemia or other conditions that lead to increased oxygen demand.

132. Answer: B) Incision into a vein—Analyze the literal meaning of phlebotomy, focusing on its

historical roots in vein incision and how it has evolved into a less invasive procedure using needles in modern medical practice.

Explanation: Phlebotomy literally means **"incision into a vein"**, derived from the Greek words "phlebo" (vein) and "tomy" (cutting). Historically, it referred to a medical practice where veins were physically cut to remove blood as part of treatments like bloodletting. In modern medicine, phlebotomy refers to the act of drawing blood using needles for diagnostic testing, blood donation, or treatment.

133. Answer: B) Decrease in cell count—Analyze the importance of "-penia" in the context of blood disorders, and explain how conditions like leukopenia or thrombocytopenia can lead to complications such as infection susceptibility or increased bleeding risk.

Explanation: The suffix **"-penia"** refers to a **decrease or deficiency** in the number of a particular type of cell, commonly used to describe conditions in the blood. For example, **leukopenia** is a reduction in white blood cells, leading to an increased risk of infections due to the body's diminished ability to fight off pathogens. **Thrombocytopenia** refers to a low platelet count, which can lead to bleeding disorders because platelets are essential for clot formation.

134. Answer: B) Fibrinolysis

Explanation: Fibrinolysis is the mechanism responsible for the breakdown of a blood clot. The enzyme **plasmin** is activated to degrade fibrin, the protein that stabilizes the clot. This process ensures that clots dissolve after they are no longer needed for wound healing, preventing thrombosis while maintaining hemostatic balance.

135. Answer: C) Phlebo-—Analyze how this prefix refers specifically to veins, as seen in terms like phlebotomy or phlebitis, and discuss its relevance in diagnostic and therapeutic procedures involving the venous system.

Explanation: The prefix **"phlebo-"** refers specifically to **veins** and is used to describe conditions and procedures related to the venous system. For example, **phlebotomy** is the process of drawing blood from a vein, while **phlebitis** is the inflammation of a vein. The use of "phlebo-" is common in both diagnostic and therapeutic contexts, especially in venous access, blood sampling, and conditions like deep vein thrombosis. While **"veno-"** also refers to veins and can sometimes

Specimen Collection and Handling

136. Answer: B) The tourniquet should be applied for no longer than 1 minute; prolonged application may lead to hemoconcentration and inaccurate test results due to falsely elevated levels of blood components.

Explanation: The tourniquet should not remain in place for more than 1 minute during venipuncture. Leaving it on longer can cause **hemoconcentration**, altering the concentration of blood cells and proteins, which may result in skewed laboratory results. If necessary, the tourniquet can be reapplied after a short rest period to allow blood flow to normalize.

137. Answer: B) 15-30 degrees, allowing the needle to enter the vein smoothly without puncturing through it, while also ensuring that the bevel is fully within the vein lumen for optimal blood flow.

Explanation: The correct needle angle for venipuncture in the antecubital space is **15 to 30 degrees**. This angle is optimal because it allows the needle to penetrate the vein at the correct depth without the risk of puncturing through the opposite wall of the vein. A steeper angle, such as 45 degrees or higher, increases the risk of going too deep or missing the vein entirely. A shallower angle, such as 5 to 10 degrees, may result in the needle slipping out of the vein, leading to unsuccessful blood collection.

Understanding and applying the correct technique, including needle angle, is essential for minimizing complications and ensuring a successful venipuncture.

138. Answer: C) Light blue top (sodium citrate)—Analyze how sodium citrate functions in coagulation studies by binding calcium and preserving coagulation factors, and why maintaining the correct blood-to-anticoagulant ratio is critical for accurate results in tests such as PT and aPTT.

Explanation: The **light blue top** tube contains **sodium citrate**, an anticoagulant that binds calcium ions, which are essential for the clotting process. This tube is specifically designed for **coagulation studies** because it prevents the blood from clotting while preserving the functionality of clotting factors for accurate measurement. Tests such as **Prothrombin Time (PT)** and **Activated Partial Thromboplastin Time (aPTT)** rely on this anticoagulant to evaluate the blood's ability to clot under controlled conditions. The proper **blood-to-**

anticoagulant ratio (9.1) must be maintained for valid test results, which is why careful collection is required.

139. Answer: B) The specimen should be labeled immediately after collection and while still in the presence of the patient, ensuring proper patient identification and preventing mix-ups.

Explanation: Labeling a specimen immediately after collection, in the presence of the patient, ensures that the specimen is correctly identified with the appropriate patient information. This step is critical in preventing errors such as mislabeling, which can lead to incorrect diagnoses or treatment.

140. Answer: B) The specimen tube is expired, or the blood has clotted in a tube meant for anticoagulation testing, which compromises test accuracy and leads to rejection.

Explanation: A blood specimen will be rejected by the laboratory under certain conditions that compromise test accuracy or validity. For instance, using an **expired tube** may result in inaccurate preservative levels, and **inappropriate clotting** in a tube intended for anticoagulated blood (such as for coagulation studies or CBCs) can ruin the sample. **Labeling errors** or missing labels can prevent proper patient identification, posing serious risks to patient safety. Even slight underfilling may be acceptable for some tests, but significant deviations in volume can lead to rejection. Proper technique in collection, handling, and labeling is essential to prevent specimen rejection and ensure reliable test results.

141. Answer: C) Using the correct needle size (21-23 gauge), allowing blood to flow gently into the collection tube, and gently inverting the tube after collection to mix the blood with anticoagulants.

Explanation: To prevent hemolysis, it's important to use the appropriate needle size to ensure proper blood flow and minimize damage to RBCs.

Allowing blood to flow gently into the tube and gently mixing the sample prevents excessive forces that can cause red blood cells to rupture.

142. Answer: C) 23-gauge; this needle size is thin enough to minimize vein damage and prevent collapse while still allowing sufficient blood flow.

Explanation: A 23-gauge needle is ideal for small or fragile veins, as it reduces the risk of vein damage or collapse during venipuncture. It provides a balance between comfort for the patient and effective blood collection.

143. Answer: A) True

Explanation: It is best practice to perform venipuncture on the arm opposite to the one with the IV to avoid contamination from IV fluids, which can affect the accuracy of lab results. If using the opposite arm is not feasible, venipuncture may be performed below (distal to) the IV site after the IV has been stopped temporarily. This helps prevent contamination and ensures more reliable test results. Drawing blood above the IV site risks contamination and should be avoided.

144. Answer: B) The side of the fingertip on the ring or middle finger, to minimize discomfort and access an area with good capillary flow.

Explanation: The **side of the fingertip** on the **ring or middle finger** is preferred for capillary collection because it has sufficient blood flow while minimizing discomfort for the patient. This area avoids the high concentration of nerve endings found in the center of the fingertip, reducing pain.

145. Answer: B) Perform the blood draw on the opposite arm (right arm), as the left arm may have impaired lymphatic drainage and increased risk of lymphedema.

Explanation: After a mastectomy, especially if lymph nodes were removed, the affected arm (in this case, the left arm) is at increased risk for **lymphedema** due to compromised lymphatic drainage. Drawing blood from this arm can trigger or worsen lymphedema, and may increase the risk of infection or other complications.

146. Answer: B) Osteomyelitis (bone infection)

Explanation: Osteomyelitis is a serious complication of heel sticks, particularly when the puncture is performed too deeply, leading to an infection of the bone. While other complications, such as hematomas and hemolysis, are possible, osteomyelitis is specifically related to improper depth during the procedure. Proper technique ensures that the puncture is superficial enough to avoid contacting bone.

147. Answer: A) True

Explanation: Hemoconcentration occurs when a tourniquet is applied for too long, causing plasma to filter out of the blood vessels and leading to a higher concentration of cells and solutes, such as red blood cells and proteins. This can affect test accuracy, especially for tests measuring electrolyte levels, glucose, or protein concentrations. In addition to skewing results, prolonged use of the tourniquet can cause patient discomfort, bruising, or even tissue damage, making it important to limit tourniquet application to under one minute.

148.Answer: C) Draw blood from the opposite arm if possible, or below the IV insertion site if an alternate site is unavailable, to prevent dilution or contamination of the sample.

Explanation: The **opposite arm** is always preferred when an IV is running, as it eliminates the risk of the blood being contaminated by IV fluids. If the opposite arm is not available, blood should be drawn **below the IV site**, ensuring that the IV fluids do not interfere with the blood draw.

149. Answer: C) Invert the tube gently 5-10 times immediately after collection, as this prevents clot formation and avoids hemolysis while ensuring thorough mixing of the blood and anticoagulant.

Explanation: Proper handling of blood collection tubes containing anticoagulants involves **gently inverting the tube 5-10 times** after collection. This ensures that the anticoagulant, such as EDTA or citrate, is thoroughly mixed with the blood sample to prevent clot formation. Vigorous shaking or too many inversions can cause **hemolysis** (the rupture of red blood cells), which compromises the integrity of the sample and can lead to inaccurate test results. Conversely, too few inversions or improper technique can result in clotting within the tube, leading to rejected specimens. Understanding and applying the correct inversion technique is crucial for reliable lab results and patient safety.

150. Answer: B) Use a butterfly needle and apply warm compresses to the arm to help dilate the veins before the draw.

Explanation: Using a **butterfly needle** is ideal for patients with difficult veins, as it provides better control and reduces the risk of damaging fragile veins. Applying **warm compresses** helps to dilate the veins, making them more prominent and easier to access.

151. Answer: C) Releasing the tourniquet before withdrawing the needle prevents hemoconcentration, which can affect analyte concentrations and lead to inaccurate test results, while also reducing the risk of hematoma formation.

Explanation: Releasing the tourniquet before the needle is withdrawn helps prevent **hemoconcentration**, a condition where prolonged pressure causes an increase in the concentration of blood components due to reduced plasma volume. This helps ensure accurate blood test results. Additionally, releasing the tourniquet reduces the risk of forming a **hematoma**, which can occur when blood leaks out of the vein into surrounding tissues after the needle is removed.

152. Answer: B) Sudden appearance of blood in the hub of the needle

Explanation: The sudden appearance of blood in the hub of the needle (referred to as "flashback") confirms that the needle is properly positioned in the vein. Other signs, such as pain at the puncture site or resistance during insertion, are not reliable indicators of successful venous access. Flashback is a critical visual cue for healthcare providers performing venipuncture.

153. Answer: A) True

Explanation: Ensuring the patient is seated in a comfortable position with their arm fully supported helps stabilize the venipuncture site and prevent patient movement, which could interfere with the procedure. If the patient is prone to fainting or dizziness, it is safer to have them lie down to prevent injury from fainting. These precautions help ensure both patient safety and the accuracy of the blood draw.

154. Answer: B) To constrict blood flow and make veins more visible—Analyze how this technique enhances vein prominence and why it is essential for successful venipuncture, considering factors such as vein anatomy and patient variability.

Explanation: The primary purpose of using a **tourniquet** during venipuncture is to **constrict venous blood flow**, which facilitates the engorgement of veins, making them more prominent and easier to locate. This is especially important in patients with challenging venous access due to factors like obesity, dehydration, or certain medical conditions.

155. Answer: A) Collect the coagulation sample first, then the serum sample

Explanation: When collecting blood samples for both coagulation studies and serum chemistry tests, the coagulation sample should be collected first. This is because coagulation tests are highly sensitive to contamination with other additives or chemicals. Collecting the coagulation sample first prevents the potential contamination of the serum sample with clotting factors. Different tubes are used for each test type, and simultaneous collection or using the same tube for both tests would not be appropriate.

156. Answer: A) True

Explanation: Using a needle that is too small can create excessive shear forces on the red blood cells, causing them to break apart (hemolyze) as they pass through the needle. Hemolysis can lead to inaccurate lab results, especially for tests involving potassium, lactate dehydrogenase (LDH), and other intracellular components. Other causes of hemolysis include vigorous shaking of the sample tube, improper collection techniques, or drawing blood from a site with excessive pressure.

157. Answer: B) To engorge the veins, making them more visible and easier to puncture for blood collection.

Explanation: The primary purpose of a tourniquet is to **engorge the veins**, enhancing their visibility and palpability for venipuncture. Proper use allows for easier access to the vein, increasing the chances of a successful blood draw.

158. Answer: B) Obtain small blood samples for testing

Explanation: Capillary tubes are primarily used to collect small blood samples, typically obtained through capillary punctures, for diagnostic tests like hemoglobin or glucose levels. They are not designed for collecting large volumes of blood, measuring arterial blood gases, or long-term storage of blood.

159. Answer: D) Gently pulling back the plunger slowly reduces turbulence during collection,

minimizing shear forces on red blood cells and thereby preventing hemolysis.

Explanation: To prevent hemolysis when using a syringe for blood collection, it is crucial to **gently pull back the plunger slowly**. This technique helps maintain a smooth flow of blood into the syringe, thereby reducing turbulence and shear stress on the red blood cells, which can cause them to rupture. Rapid withdrawal (A) can introduce significant turbulence, leading to hemolysis. While larger bore needles (B) may facilitate smoother blood flow, using an appropriate gauge needle in conjunction with slow withdrawal is the best practice. Proper angling (C) is important for access, but maintaining a gentle technique throughout the collection process is key to preserving sample integrity and ensuring accurate laboratory results.

160. Correct Answer: B) The patient is a pediatric patient with small veins, and the phlebotomist anticipates a need for precise control during the blood collection.

Explanation: Using a **butterfly needle** is ideal for patients with **small, fragile veins** where precision and control are critical. The design of the butterfly needle allows for easier access and minimizes trauma to the vein.